And Other Duties as Assigned

And Other Duties as Assigned

WALKING THE PATH OF A CHAPLAIN MANAGER INSIDE AND OUTSIDE THE WALLS

REV. GRAYLIN CARLTON
Chaplain Manager, FaithHealth and Chaplaincy Ministries, Atrium Health Wake Forest Baptist-Wilkes Medical Center in North Wilkesboro, NC

REV. DIANNE HORTON
Manager, Chaplaincy and Clinical Ministries, Atrium Health Wake Forest Baptist-Lexington Medical Center in Lexington, NC

REV. DR. ADAM RIDENHOUR
Manager, Chaplaincy and Clinical Ministries, Atrium Health Wake Forest Baptist Davie Medical Center, a division of NC Baptist Hospital, in Bermuda Run, NC

REV. DR. EMILY VIVERETTE
Director of FaithHealth Chaplaincy and Education, Atrium Health Wake Forest Baptist in Winston-Salem, NC

With MELANIE RASKIN

Copyright © 2025 by Stakeholder Press
All rights reserved. No parts of this book may be reproduced or used in any manner without written permission of the copyright owner except for use of quotations in the book.

   Stakeholder Press
   www.hold.health

The contents of this book represent the views of the authors and not Atrium Health Wake Forest Baptist.

ISBN: 978-1-7324222-7-8

Project director: Tom Peterson

Cover and book design: H. K. Stewart

Stakeholder Press
BOOKS TO MAKE THE WORLD BETTER

Printed in the United States of America

Table of Contents

1. Introduction... 7

2. The FaithHealth Chaplaincy Model: A Framework
   for Caring... 21

3. Who We Are: Roles and Responsibilities 37

4. For the Good of the Hive: Community Engagement 53

5. Nailing Jello to the Wall: Measuring the Impact of
   Chaplain Managers 73

6. Anglers and Bakers: Core Competencies and Skills 89

7. The Cup that Runneth Over: Challenges, Lessons,
   The Future... 105

References 129

About the Authors 139

1.
Introduction

Health is a state of complete physical, mental, and social well-being and not merely the absence of disease or infirmity.
— World Health Organization (WHO)

"Being a chaplain manager enables me to capitalize on my connections, my expertise, and my compassion to get patients where they need to go."
— Graylin Carlton

When the call came, Graylin Carlton knew just what to do. The veteran on the phone needed help. Sick with cancer and bleeding badly, the man had to get to the VA hospital two hours away in Asheville, North Carolina, but he lived alone and had no car. Carlton arranged transportation so the veteran could be driven to the hospital and admitted into the care he needed. It all happened quickly, easily, and efficiently. That's because Carlton had written the grant for the transportation program that drove the mostly rural county patients without rides to their medical appointments.

Graylin Carlton isn't a social worker. He's not a health care provider. He isn't the veteran's buddy, nor is he a volunteer in a nonprofit. Yet, on the other hand, he is *all* those things. Rev. Graylin Carlton is Chaplain Manager at Atrium Health Wake Forest Baptist-Wilkes Medical Center in North Wilkesboro, North Carolina, a healthcare facility serving the mostly rural population of Wilkes County. Graylin Carlton and chaplain managers like him do this every day. They minister to patients in every way—from the spiritual to the corporeal—with a focus on ensuring people get the health care they need and deserve.

Unfortunately, the veteran's story is a familiar one. According to the American Hospital Association, every year 3.6 million people miss out on medical services due to transportation problems.[1] For older patients, lack of access to a vehicle is the third most common barrier to health care. A 2020 study published in the American Journal of Public Health found that the patients most affected by transportation barriers to health care were those who were poor or experiencing chronic conditions.[2]

Fortunately, Chaplain Graylin Carlton's story is becoming The New Normal. It is a story of empowerment—for the patient *and* for him. Chaplain managers work inside *and outside* the walls of the hospital to remove barriers to care. It's a tightrope they walk, but they are trained to keep one foot in the institutional world of the hospital and the other foot in the real world of their small, rural community. More importantly, because of who they are at their core and what they do, they are willing (and more crucially, *able*), as Dr. Martin Luther King, Jr., advised, to take that first step even when they can't see the whole staircase.

Stepping Into the Gap: What Are Chaplain Managers?

> *"A chaplain manager is a great addition to smaller and rural hospitals with fewer than a hundred beds across the country. Oftentimes these institutions don't have staff chaplains. This model makes the case for adding one because it expands the role in new and creative ways."*
>
> — Emily Viverette

Chaplain managers are the personification of the national FaithHealth movement, a program dedicated to improving health by getting people to the right door at the right time, ready to be treated, and not alone. And no, it's not a typo. The words "Faith" and "Health" are intentionally joined by the movement's founder Rev. Gary Gunderson, author, teacher, public health thought leader, and former health care executive. He states that in some African languages, as well as in Aramaic, the native language of Jesus and ancient Middle Eastern cultures, the notions of faith and health cannot—*should not*—be separated.[3] These ancient cultures instinctively knew—and still know today—that spiritual care, medical care, community health, counseling, and the health of congregations are tightly—*and rightly*—bound together.[4]

FaithHealth activates its mission of healing through dynamic working partnerships between health systems, faith communities, and organizations and nonprofits focused on enhancing the health and well-being of body, mind, and spirit. Expertly uniting the heart for service of congregations, the clinical expertise of health care providers, and the in-the-trenches offerings and resources of local networks and agencies is the job—*the calling*—of chaplain managers.

But what chaplain managers are *not* is equally important. The necessity for skilled and trained chaplain managers arises from the challenges of providing bio-psycho-social-spiritual care within healthcare settings, particularly in rural and small communities. Hospitals in these remote regions often rely on untrained volunteers for support. While the intentions of volunteers may be genuine, the lack of formal education and training can lead to unintended spiritual distress for patients. Some volunteers may use their position to further personal agendas, such as spiritual recruitment for their congregation or financial gain through services such as funeral arrangements. Chaplain managers won't leverage a patient or relationship. They aren't recruiting congregation members, they will not seek business or profit, they don't have personal agendas. They are hired and trained professional members of the hospital team tasked with providing compassionate spiritual care, in the moment, from the patient's spiritual perspective. Their job? To meet patients where they are.

While chaplain managers serve the traditional role as the hospital's spiritual care professionals, they are unique in the chaplaincy realm. That's because of the broad scope of the FaithHealth mission. Bottom line, their work is all about healing communities—both within and outside the hospital. The role is crucial, but it is often complicated and always nuanced.

Chaplain managers:

- Deliver spiritual care to patients, as well as hospital colleagues,
- Work within the hospital system to improve institutional processes and access to care,
- Provide 24/7 crisis response for patients and hospital staff,
- Partner with local community agencies to share or create needed resources and programs to support whole-person health, and
- Team up with faith communities to activate the FaithHealth mission of accompanying patients on their health journeys.

It's a tall order—and not for the faint-hearted. Being a chaplain manager takes education, trust, expertise, compassion, courage, and of course, faith. And not just Christian faith. While the authors of this book are immersed in Christian culture because of their service areas in North Carolina, they have expertise working across many religious traditions. It's an integral part of the FaithHealth chaplaincy paradigm to understand that effective chaplaincy comes from *all* faith walks. There's a reason what we know as The Golden Rule appears not just in Christian culture but also in most other major religious culture, as well as ancient Greek and Egyptian texts. "Do unto others as you would have them do unto you" are profound words to live by—and a foundational precept of effective chaplaincy. That concept knows no geographical borders, no lines in the sand, no religious divisions. That's the true beauty of the FaithHealth model of chaplaincy. It is fully embedded in its community and true to the roots of the culture in which it exists and serves. Chaplain managers are not just Jewish or Christian, Muslim or Buddhist, Hindu or Bahá'í followers, Shintoists or Taoists. They are people assiduously trained to meet others where they are, lifting up the stories, values, and perspectives of the people they journey with, regardless of backgrounds and faith traditions.

"I think about safe space: providing safe space for others and finding safe space for myself."
— Dianne Horton

"Cultural humility is part of the safe space and adaptability. You've got to be humble to adapt."
— Emily Viverette

HOLDING THE SPACE

Dianne Horton's teammate at the Lexington Medical Center was very sick. The patient's medical provider was ready to move heaven and earth to perform a medical procedure with only a small chance of helping for a short time ... but the patient refused. She did not want any intervention—she was good with where she was on her life journey. Horton, as Chaplain Manager, was called in to be a part of the conversation, to help the doctor and patient really hear each other. "The real gift as a chaplain manager is that I am neutral," she said. "I'm here to facilitate the conversation. Yes, I have my opinions, but it's not my role to share what I would do in a given situation. It's all about the patient. I'm here to support the patient's autonomy to make her own decisions."

Different from Traditional Chaplains

Traditional chaplaincy in a hospital focuses primarily on the one-on-one experience, family unit care, teammate encounter, or ritual leadership during the work day. But in a world where chaplains aren't the only people providing spiritual care anymore, FaithHealth has evolved the model to something wider and different. Because of a conscious move from a siloed structure to a partnership paradigm, the FaithHealth chaplaincy model includes not only the traditional chaplaincy duties of ministering to patients, families, and staff of the hospital but also community engagement and, when appropriately credentialed, counseling. This inevitably—and intentionally—leads to a more upstream approach and big picture system, with the focus on prevention, holistic care, increasing access to care by reducing barriers and addressing social drivers of health, and getting patients to the right door at the right time, ready to be treated and never alone.

Another critical but subtle difference from traditional chaplaincy is that chaplain managers are specialists precisely trained to partner with community generalists to provide care both inside *and* outside the hospital. It's a bold approach, but it makes sense: After all, most of a patient's life is spent outside the walls of the healthcare facility. The chaplain manager role evolves the standard nine-to-five spiritual care day helmed by a sole practitioner within the hospital to a twenty-four/seven system of whole-person support that follows patients wherever they go. The truth is, most people experiencing spiritual care in a community nowadays never see traditional clergy or congregation.[5] Spiritual care is bigger, more organic, and open now—dynamics FaithHealth was built for and, in many ways, helped launch.

"It's not an either-or. This model is an expansion, an extension."
— Emily Viverette

"One important dynamic for me is that it's starting to all run together. I know what lane I need to be in as a chaplain manager in a hospital policy-related issue. But in terms of the care I provide, so much of that and the theory I operate from is informed by the fact that a patient may be calling for prayer but it could be a social driver or access issue they're dealing with. Or maybe the anxiety has popped up because of the psychotropic drugs the person is on. Whatever it is, the interconnectedness of all of it is very clear to me—I'm more attuned to that now than ever."
— Adam Ridenhour

> "Before when I was in a traditional chaplaincy department, it felt siloed. But now, I'm not separated; I'm a bigger part of what goes on in the hospital. My hospital leader will come to me and share what's going on and ask my opinion about how to approach things. I like that, I like the flexibility in my role. Being part of the bigger picture is meaningful and satisfying."
> — Graylin Carlton

Why This Model? Why Now?

Change is happening at lightning speed in small and rural communities as local nonprofit hospitals are acquired in medical system mergers.[6,7] Smaller hospitals in big networks can suffer because resources are often more heavily focused on the larger campuses.[6,7] Small communities have watched key medical units shut down after mergers, with the resulting loss of or change in medical staff.[6,7] The Lexington Medical Center in North Carolina closed its labor and delivery unit when the bigger system they are a part of opened a major birthing center. But it's a both-and situation. While there may be a loss of local services, there can also be the benefits of a larger system with more technology and resources on offer. Change is also an integral part of the hospital's Community Health Needs Assessment (CHNA), a tool that helps the healthcare system improve the overall health and well-being of its community, including biological, social, psychological, and spiritual wellness.

In these small and rural hospitals where community ties are close and binding, having a professional chaplain manager as a strategic partner to help navigate change and implement the hospital's CHNA strategies proves particularly advantageous. Living and working in these rural areas translates into an intimate understanding of the local culture, which enhances sensitivity to and awareness of the needs of patients, and so, of the broader community. Because of the smaller size of the hospitals and communities they traditionally serve, chaplain managers become a representative of the medical center. They work with patients as they weave in and out of the system, ensuring that health is not restricted to just the hospital building but is a vibrant part of the tapestry of the community.

An important part of that flow is assessing and shining a light on how care is divided by socioeconomic status, gender issues, racial divisions, and more, and then challenging those systems of injustice that foster division and separation in the community—both inside and outside the hospital setting. Chaplain managers help hospitals understand how to be better neighbors in their communities by standing firmly in the middle and serving as a conduit between the two, educating and guiding the trusting community to the hospital to be served. It is a holistic approach to health that aligns smoothly with the chaplain manager's expertise. And it works. Because chaplain managers are respectful companions on whatever healing journey the patient is on (providing spiritual care, ensuring opportunities for access to health care, and serving as advocates to remove barriers to care), they are part of the fabric of their community. Think denim: durable, resilient, and comfortable.

The chaplain manager model is crucial to communities now, not only to improve overall health but also to save patients, the hospital, and other support systems money by getting people to the right door at the right time, ready to be treated. This proven model enhances quality of life and can even extend life. And along the way, it gives people dignity as they walk their health care path, ensuring patients are truly heard and getting the access to the services they need.

> *"We are a voice for the voiceless. Not everybody has a seat at the table and it's a privilege to have the seat we hold."*
> — Dianne Horton

BUILDING BRIDGES

When Graylin Carlton first came to Wilkes Medical Center as Chaplain Manager, there were people who would not come to the hospital, due to generations-deep, racially-based, and completely understandable mistrust, fear, and suspicion. That's different now, years later. "I feel like I've been a conduit in the community," he said. "I'm doing my work and now everyone in our community feels like they can come to the hospital and be served. It wasn't like that before; the lack of a chaplain in the community was detrimental. Having a chaplain has helped build those bridges and restore trust."

Challenges Beget Opportunities

The work of a chaplain manager comes with challenges and opportunities. The challenges are what you'd expect in a role that is focused on service and people: time and money. In this era of shrinking healthcare resources, it can be hard to demonstrate financial value to a hospital's bottom line, much less identify the metrics to evaluate a chaplain manager's contributions. And when you can't demonstrate value in black and white on a spreadsheet, it makes it tough to get needed resources of funding or additional personnel. On the other hand, the hospital system mergers that result from those shrinking healthcare resources are creating opportunities to ensure that the most vulnerable patients don't fall through the cracks, thanks to multiple networks and more service offerings.

Another challenge is the unknown. Chaplain managers are often thrown into situations with a clean slate and mandated to figure out what's going on and how to help. Conversely, the unknown is also an opportunity to get creative. Because the slate is blank, chaplain managers are free to explore new ideas and try new things. However, the increasing corporatization of the healthcare world and its mandate to systemize processes, procedures, and even people can result in the restriction of freedom. The new opportunity? Get *even more* creative.

And then there's the identity crisis: Chaplain managers wear two hats in the hospital. They are part of the hospital management system *and* its support system. There's tension in serving both the institution and the people at the same time. But there's also a beautiful expansiveness—a stretch that benefits both the patient and the hospital. Chaplain managers' deep knowledge of the hospital system means they intimately understand oftentimes complex processes and can bring real wisdom and insider expertise to people in need of spiritual care. And because they are trained chaplains, they can help the hospital humanize, and so, improve those processes.

Sometimes, relationships are challenging. It can be hard for hospitals and communities to see eye-to-eye. Chaplain managers are smack-dab in the middle of what can often feel like a tug of war. Being in the middle is a unique and exciting position, full of possibilities. One possibility-turned-reality that perfectly matches the role and skills of chaplain managers is the requirement of the Affordable Care Act (ACA) for nonprofit hospitals to provide "community benefit."[8] The value chaplain managers bring to the community benefit aspect of the hospital's work delivers a significant return on investment for both the hospital and the community because it fuels creativity in community leaders and captures the attention of healthcare executives. Because their job has chaplain managers out in the community where they can see and hear about the need for improvement, they know what has to shift to enhance care and improve lives. But it's also a compromised position, because they are within the systems of an institution that can be hard to budge. But, when it moves, it's amazing—and profoundly impactful.

A Powerful Why

The work of chaplain managers in smaller hospitals makes a strong case for spiritual care as an ally in the new norm of value-based health care. Chaplain managers are integral in the mission of ensuring healthy people stay healthy by being that important advocate within—*and outside*—the walls of the hospital, aligning resources to help patients access their medicines, make regular appointments with doctors instead of coming through the emergency department, and get the food, shelter, and transportation they need.

In the case of chaplain mangers, size matters. It is because of the size of their communities that chaplain managers are in the unique position to unite the training, the capacity, the history, the connections, and the relationships to deliver *true* care and *real* support. In small and rural hospitals, chaplain managers are able to deliver authentic, compassionate spiritual care because they are brave enough and bold enough to plant a foot in both worlds—the hospital's and the community's—and see where the path leads.

THE CASE FOR CHAPLAIN MANAGERS

It's all about healthy communities. From the financial perspective, professional chaplain managers save money and put resources where they belong, aligning with the goals of Medicare and Medicaid. "The nation's healthcare system is very complex and hard to navigate," said Adam Ridenhour. "Having trusted people that the community can reach out to can help. Being the resource, the bridge, is The Why for many people entering this field. We're here to help people navigate this complicated system and come out the other side feeling empowered and truly supported."

"We have the opportunity in the size hospitals we're in and the communities we serve to be extensions of the medical center. It's our job to follow patients as they come in and as they leave, ensuring health is not just a fixture of the hospital building but part of the tapestry of the community."

— Adam Ridenhour

"This approach has been a part of the role of churches and chaplains in smaller communities for a long time. Our model formally empowers our chaplain managers to seek out this work and do it, to make it more visible and a part of the workday."

— Emily Viverette

"This work has been done before by others; it's just not called this by others."

— Dianne Horton

2.

The FaithHealth Chaplaincy Model:
A Framework for Caring

"Ministry is ministry. It's helping people, it's putting self aside and doing what's right. Chaplaincy in a rural county, it makes sense to go outside the hospital."

— Graylin Carlton

"I'm motivated by faith—being able to accompany people on their journeys as well as hold opposing things together. On a more practical basis, the work we do is impacting patient care by emphasizing holistic care in ways it has not been before, from fee-for-service to population health. Yes, we are affecting patients in front of us now in good ways, and we are doing upstream work as well in helping to define what supportive, spiritual care will look like ten years from now. This work is innovative."

— Adam Ridenhour

"I think one of the meanings of salvation is wholeness."

— Dianne Horton

We all know the standard health metrics assessing wellness: temperature, blood pressure, blood type, sugar level, cholesterol, etc. But in his research, Adam Ridenhour cited other equally important factors that affect health that are harder to measure and yet are also universal across all populations. These include access to health care, affordability of care, healthy foods and clean drinking water, safe shelter, and supportive mental health.[9] These social drivers of health are not egalitarian—as always, some people have and others have not. Ridenhour also pointed out that health care issues are mired in webs of systems. Yes, diet and exercise are foundational to cardiovascular health, but so are the more subtle points of access to that healthy food and regular exercise, the ability to schedule and get to consistent physicals with medical doctors and dentists, and the impacts of stress and substances such as tobacco, alcohol, and drugs. These factors don't just affect the individual; they also shape communities.[9]

It's the inextricable web of these factors and their significant impact on people that are behind the basic framework of the FaithHealth model. Founded by author, teacher, public health thought leader, and health care executive Rev. Gary Gunderson in Memphis, Tennessee, more than twenty years ago, it is currently expanding into hospitals in other states. The premise of FaithHealth is simple, yet profound: to understand that most of people's lives are lived in their community; therefore, logically, most health and healing happen *outside* the walls of the hospital. Because estimates attest that medical care accounts for only 10 to 20 percent of health outcomes,[10,11] FaithHealth is an integrated approach to holistic care designed to expand the patient's health care journey beyond the walls of the hospital and out into the community, saving the hospital and patients money, especially the higher costs of delayed treatment for medical conditions-turned-crises.[12] Supporting people, especially the underserved, by reducing barriers and increasing access to care effectively improves not only individual health but also community health, ultimately saving lives.[12]

CHAPLAIN MANAGEMENT 101: SPEAKING TRUTH TO POWER

Chaplain managers are bioethics champions; champions of diversity, equity, and inclusion; champions for patient relations and the experience of patients who walk through the hospital's doors; champions of a family-centered environment. That means their care isn't limited to the medical research community's traditional "model patient": the relatively healthy and well-resourced person with an uncomplicated life history and no known comorbidities, who doesn't smoke or drink, who meditates an hour a day, who does all the right things that lead to health, who can champion their own health care—*and* has health insurance. While that is the picture-perfect way health systems are currently designed to function, chaplain managers operate in the real world with real patients, outside of the fairy tale 'norms.' A uniqueness of the job is the way they live their commitment to equality and equity through action. "We predominantly work with folks whose voices are not heard on the same level and platform that other patients are," Adam Ridenhour said. "Our job—our duty—is to make an impact on that person's life. It may be as simple as helping them apply for Medicaid and lining up transportation so they can turn in their paperwork. That's a good day."

That's the principal difference between chaplain managers and traditional chaplains. Chaplain managers are tasked with activating the FaithHealth model in their communities: building a steadfast and action-oriented corps of congregations, healthcare system, and community people and agencies to get patients to the right door at the right time, ready to be treated. They integrate chaplaincy and community engagement—and some bring licensed counseling skills to the table—to improve individual and community health, especially for the marginalized. This union of the spiritual with the managerial, inspirational with the tactical, faith with works, requires a different way of being and an expanded set of skills beyond traditional chaplaincy, including entrepreneurship, flexibility, adaptability, and creativity.

However, the corporatization of health care, which relies on the systemization of, well, just about everything, leaves less room for those skills. Yet nothing demands entrepreneurship, flexibility, adaptability, and creativity more than the new paradigm of value-based health care. All of these skills begin with freedom, which can feel diametrically opposed to an organization that lives and dies by a rigorously designed and assiduously implemented set of often complex, narrowly defined systems. There's a natural tension in how chaplain managers deploy their skills. On the one hand, they are hired to be advocates and create change, but on the other hand, they are working within systems that are difficult to change. It's a big ask to shift a culture from solely focusing on inside the walls of the hospital to a broader and greater vision of treating the whole person wherever they are on their healing path, including in their daily lives out in the community. How do chaplain managers walk this path? How do they perform their expansive, broad-based work in a more confined, highly regulated industry?

Being part of a team helps. Chaplain managers work with contract on-call chaplain associates, administrative assistants, and connectors. Connectors are lightly funded bridge-builders, networkers, and advocates who live in and know the community and provide hands-on caregiving, such as delivering meals and medicines, dropping by for visits, and recruiting and training volunteers. Connectors make excellent partners because some are already embedded in local networks, such as denominations and faith-based agencies, and can leverage their affiliations to activate resources for patients and community members. Because an important part of their work is community engagement, chaplain managers are also part of teams of willing, tireless, inspired activists, organizations, churches, and ordinary citizens dedicated to the common goal of health and well-being for all. There are two guiding principles that are crucial to the work: leading causes of life and boundary leadership.

Leading Causes of Life

We've all heard the phrase, the only sure thing is death and taxes. There *is* one other sure thing: *life*. There is no death without life (and there certainly aren't taxes without it!). The Leading Causes of Life Initiative was developed by Gary Gunderson, creator of the FaithHealth model, former Vice President for Faith and Health at Atrium Health Wake Forest Baptist Medical Center, and Professor of Public Health Sciences and Professor of Religion and the Health of the Public at Wake Forest University School of Divinity, and James Cochrane. This perspective shifts the community's institutionalized health care focus on problem-solving from that which harms us (leading causes of death) to those things that work for us—that expansive, innovative energy of life that benefits not only the individual but also the community. The leading causes of life are agency, coherence, connection, intergenerativity (blessing), and hope.[13,14] They guide not only the mindsets but also the problem-solving work of chaplain managers in their communities.

LEADING CAUSE OF LIFE: AGENCY

This is the capacity for creative freedom: to act intentionally in the world with the moral awareness of our responsibility for what, how, and why we do things. It is innate, ephemeral yet real, and absolutely central to who we are as human beings. This is the power, will, and resourcefulness to *do*, to rise above "what is" and birth new possibilities—whether it's to build a new vacuum cleaner, create a beautiful sculpture, or launch an innovative transportation initiative that drives people without access to a vehicle to their doctor's appointment.[13,14]

LEADING CAUSE OF LIFE: COHERENCE

Coherence is how we make sense of life and bring order, intelligence, and a sense of purpose to our experiences along the life journey. Instead of randomness and victimhood, coherence includes the ability to thrive, resilience, coping, meaning-making, and adaptation.[13,14]

LEADING CAUSE OF LIFE: CONNECTION

According to Gunderson, without connection there is no community, and without community there is no life. Whether it's meeting the basic human needs for food, water, and shelter; enhancing prestige; or inspiring creative freedom to the highest level of achievement, connection finds life through building relationships with each other and building communities that help us meet ever-evolving challenges and opportunities. Spanning across family, friends, and community, this includes social capital, connectedness, and involvement.[13,14]

LEADING CAUSE OF LIFE: INTERGENERATIVITY

Also termed *blessing*, intergenerativity centers on approval, affirmation, support, encouragement, nurturing, strengthening, praising, mentoring, teaching, being a positive influence, and beholding the sacredness of others. It's namaste: the divine in me bows to the divine in you. Blessing empowers us to make important choices that shape our own lives and live up to our potential—not just for our highest and best good but for the well-being of those around us as well. It's the ability to become something better. In communities, it's a collective choice.[13,14]

Leading Cause of Life: Hope

In Jesus's time, the Hebrew and native Aramaic word for "hope" was powerful. It meant "confidently expecting," "to trust and wait expectantly."[15,16,17] As a leading cause of life, it wields the same authority *and* promise for all people of all faith walks around the globe. More than optimism and wishful thinking, hope is our ability to imagine a different, healthier future and, equally important, to marshal the energy, will, and intention to cocreate that future—to birth something new and better.[15,16,17] As Gunderson wrote, "Hope consists in our trust that it is never possible for us to lose Spirit and our spiritual capacities so long as we are alive."[13,14] Hope is the trust in who and what we are, and that new possibilities always lie before us, whether we can achieve them or not. Hope inspires individual and collective action. The chaplain manager's capacity to focus on possibilities, meaning, relationships, and empowerment leads them to search for life and hope in areas where others see only need and despair.[13,14]

Boundary Leadership

An important part of a chaplain manager's calling to be a catalyst for change that supports health and well-being for all, including the underserved, is boundary leadership: seeing boundaries as relationships to build and possibilities to lift up instead of silos to protect and territories to defend. This is equally exciting and frightening, lonely and connecting, spiritual and structural—often at the same time. FaithHealth founder Gary Gunderson's seminal proposition is that congregations should be expanding their vision to include engaging with the challenges affecting a community's most vulnerable citizens, a twenty-first century version of the vibrant public interest service role faith communities played in early American history. Gunderson's mind-opening philosophy sees boundaries as the edges of where things join instead of the places where things separate.[9] But this way of being comes with challenges. Boundary leaders can feel lonely and out of their depth because they're out of their wheelhouse and in new territory. It can be hard meeting new people and building new, different relationships outside of the reliable and easy comfort zone of the usual friends, family, church, and traditional chaplaincy role of the workplace.[18]

Gunderson states boundary leaders "align the assets of community with the most relevant science and most mature faith." They have the courage and optimism to identify broken systems and then seek out and focus on areas of the community centered on life, working with community strategic partners to leverage that empowering, healing energy broad-scale to repair failed systems and enhance quality of life in every significant measure for every person: health and hope, abundance and prosperity, love and connection, and peace and harmony.[9]

The five characteristics of boundary leadership include the ability to read reality, see "the whole" of a situation, and embrace the complexity of people and systems. Boundary leaders live with misunderstanding because their work for the greater good is often seen as out of bounds—the very definition of boundary leadership is to view boundaries as opportunities for unity and growth instead of division and stasis. Boundary leaders build bridges—and work to keep them open, linking people with different viewpoints, talents, and energies in the service of creating greater beneficial change. They weave networks or webs for transformation, creating organic structures that can evolve with the community for real, sustainable, long-term success. Last, boundary leaders actively counter the negative valence by seeking and holding the positive valence.

When disparities, dehumanization, and damage occur in a community, fear and negativity abound—from the wounded *and* from those systems doing the wounding. Expectations can be unrealistic. Boundary leaders turn around the negative valence by holding and shining the light of the positive valence until all can see and trust it, pulling together the disparate broken pieces into one stable, evolving whole for the well-being of all.[18]

Boundary leaders walk the talk. They are smack in the middle of the reality of the community they are actively engaged with on the journey to positive transformation, with an unswerving and courageous focus always on people, communities, and relationships and how they are hurt or healed.[18]

> *"It can be difficult seeing the ministry in the administrative pieces of the job because that seems to be the greatest piece of the job: looking at policies, procedures, guidelines, and budgets through that lens of justice. Are we doing the things that God would have us to do and being a voice to that?"*
> — Dianne Horton

BOUNDARY LEADERSHIP: A DOUBLE-EDGED SWORD

Because of deep and humble listening, connecting with his community, meeting patients where they are, and earning trust, Graylin Carlton was able to improve access to his hospital's cancer center so that fewer people missed their appointments, improving health and possibly even saving lives. But, it raised some eyebrows. Carlton was doing his job of solidifying the connection with the community as mandated by the hospital, and at the same time it could be interpreted that he was bucking a carefully created system that didn't have a line item or process for that type of active invitation to community people with health issues. "Sometimes it can feel like we're doing something wrong and are breaking one of the rules, that we're out of compliance with the standards of the hospital," he said. "My hope is that we come up with a way for the system to understand what we do and how it fits in with the hospital's mission to support the health of the community. Everything we do is because we're chaplains and we care for the people we serve. I could never go to another board meeting, never sit down in another grant meeting to raise money to help people, never arrange transportation for another patient to get to the doctor again, but my community would suffer for it—and ultimately, so would the hospital."

A Framework for Caring

"Health and wellness feed into theology, having a desire to see people whole in every way. FaithHealth is about ministering to a person's whole being."

— Adam Ridenhour

"The reality is we shouldn't need chaplains. We should be trying to work ourselves out of jobs. But, people need chaplains because many don't have the spiritual and emotional support they need. There are communication challenges, there are systems challenges, there are other things happening. If the health system truly works for all, if every healthcare provider in the institution had the time and space for deep listening with patients and families and accompanying them through crises, we wouldn't need chaplains. We are here to help bridge gaps in holistic care and provide spiritual support for those who need it."

— Emily Viverette

All of these frames of reference and ways of being are important touchstones—even beacons—on the chaplain manager's walk along what they see as the inextricable conjoined edges of the former boundaries of the medical center and the community it serves. Yet none of these models are as important as heart, courage, and a stalwart commitment—many would say sacred call—to step into the gap and assure just and fair access to care for the most vulnerable people during times of growing economic and health disparities. To help others is not a bullet point that regularly shows up on job descriptions, which makes it an irresistible invitation for those who are instinctively built to do good in the world.

Adam Ridenhour finds the chaplain manager ethos in the Christian story in the fifth chapter of the Gospel of Luke: the miracle of Jesus healing the paralyzed man. In the story, there is such a crowd surrounding Jesus that friends could not bring the sick man lying on his mat close enough for healing. So instead, these good neighbors climbed up on the roof and lowered him through the ceiling tiles right in front of Jesus in the middle of the crowd. According to Luke, when Jesus witnessed their faith, he forgave the man's sins and commanded him to stand and walk. According to Ridenhour, chaplain managers are the neighbors in this story, fortified by faith, compassion, and a sense of justice to get people the care they need.[9]

Lifting Up Community Assets to Meet Local Needs

Asset-mapping, the process of building a community from the inside out,[19,20] revealed several key needs in Davie County, NC: a lack of public transportation, the absence of behavioral health providers, and a disconnect between faith communities and nonprofits providing services. More importantly, it also revealed invaluable resources and capacities: a number of churches and food banks were willing to distribute food if they knew there was an opportunity for partnership. In another case, stretched-thin mental health professionals and pediatric clinicians were unaware that local congregations wanted to help address high suicide and infant mortality rates. What was left after the asset map was to connect the dots and start the conversation.[9] One conversation led to a chaplain manager and FaithHealth leaders traveling to Liberty, NC, to explore a community transportation model that addressed some of the same needs Davie County was facing. The result? The birth of The Last Mile, a Davie County nonprofit focused on providing transportation to promote health and wholeness. This initiative that helps people get to medical appointments, grocery stores, and other day-to-day activities was founded by a FaithHealth connector and local pastor, and is based on the program in Liberty. "This ministry model addresses the need for transportation in our community and exemplifies the FaithHealth logic of leading causes of life and boundary leadership," Adam Ridenhour said. "At the same time, it lifts up the assets of a local faith community, volunteers, local and national funding, and denominational support. Asset-mapping is an important part of our work."

Guiding Frameworks: A Definition of Terms

While leading causes of life and boundary leadership inform the chaplain manager ways of being, there are other key practices, theories, and frameworks that chaplain managers look to for guidance, including:

Abundance Mindset vs. Scarcity Mindset

The brainchild of business guru and author Steven Covey in his 1989 book, *The Seven Habits of Highly Effective People*, abundance mindset is the belief that there is more than enough of everything for everyone: plentiful resources, opportunity, and success. The scarcity mindset, which can come from true scarcity, is a win-lose proposition, a viewpoint that's all about limits and a world of "not enough"—not enough money, not enough time, not enough love, not enough hope, not enough help for everyone. People with an abundance mindset see life as a win-win for all, with endless possibilities. Individuals with a scarcity mindset feel like their share of resources and opportunities will always be limited and others will always have more.[21,22]

Asset-Based World View

An asset-based world view goes hand-in-hand with an abundance mindset. In the health care arena, the traditional medical model and ways of working are rooted in disease state and processes—spring-boarding from what's wrong or damaged in an individual or a community. An asset-based point of view sees the community as the key to long-lasting, meaningful change. This grassroots-focused lens on the world builds on the desires, gifts, and strengths of local citizens, organizations and nonprofits, and institutions to mobilize sustainable change that promote long-term wholeness and well-being.[12,19]

Asset-Mapping

Asset-mapping is the procedure that gives legs to an asset-based lens. This process can reveal the need for new initiatives and services, as well as support decision-making. Asset-mapping is a form of walking the talk focused on uncovering and leveraging a community's current resources (people power, buildings, policies, businesses, and funding) instead of getting mired in the needs. This process achieves community development goals by formally identifying the strengths, gifts, talents, skills, capacities, and resources of local individuals, associations (groups and organizations), and entities (government, education, health care, human services) to meet needs and achieve important common goals.[20,23]

Positive Deviance

The premise of positive deviance is that the best way to solve tough problems is to look to local wisdom and emulate people who have succeeded in facing down the same issues, against the odds. It's an asset-based, community-driven approach to problem-solving that brings people together to find those winning strategies and behaviors and adapt them into an action plan for the current challenge.[24]

Living Human Web

Fundamental to contemporary pastoral theology, the living human web stretches the chaplain's capacity to empathize by broadening the traditional focus from a strictly spiritual or religious purview to a wider social and cultural context. This opens the conversation and expands understanding to include examining the impacts of social injustice and the challenges facing people in need by including more and diverse voices (women, people of color, LGBTQ+, etc.).[25]

Failing Systems Theory

Systems fail when obsolete models fail. For example, the breaking down of complicated public policy problems into seemingly simpler individual parts, and the resulting ever-growing complexity of interactions and blurred boundaries, can conclude in an inability to meet the challenges communities face. It's not so much a failure of the parts but rather the links between the parts. No longer linear, this complex web of human, technology, policy, communication, and program interconnections makes it much harder to figure out what went wrong and why, and nearly impossible to predict future failure.[26] As systems become more complicated, open communication and feedback, diverse input from a number of voices—even the unlikeliest, and transparency are vital.[27]

Structuralism

Structuralism is a methodology that sees the world through structures. Predominant in the social sciences, structuralism posits that things cannot be understood in isolation, but rather only in the context of broader systems. It boils down the complexity of human culture to universal underlying systems and focuses on how these social, cultural, and psychological constructs dictate human behavior, endeavoring to reveal the patterns that undergird what people perceive, think, feel, and do.[28,29]

3.

Who We Are:
Roles and Responsibilities

"We are the face of the hospital in the world."
— Graylin Carlton

"We bring a moral spiritual compass to everything we do—from providing pastoral care support to patients and families, to connecting people in need to resources, to reviewing a hospital budget. Looking at things through the lens of fairness and justice is always a good thing."
— Dianne Horton

"I love it, walking into the unknown and the immediacy of service. There's never a boring day."
— Adam Ridenhour

Chaplain Manager Graylin Carlton's Roots

"I was looking at chaplaincy because I knew there was more to ministry than being a pastor in a rural community. I didn't want to have to watch people with alcoholism, addiction, and mental health issues die, and not be able to really help. So for me, the calling is social, it's spiritual, it's about economics, and it has a lot to do with me being a Black man. I grew up in Wilkes County and I know firsthand that the Black community did not have the resources the white community had. I watched my aunt go back and forth to the mental institution for shock treatment and die. I have watched so many die of alcoholism and there was no one there to talk to them, to help them, to give them direction. That's why I'm here, but it was a hard decision. I moved away and had no intention of returning. I decided, if I'm going back, I want *everyone* in this community to have the same resources and access as people do in bigger hospital communities. For me, it's all about access. And we did it: Now Wilkes has a cardiac rehab heart center; we've expanded our emergency department (ED) services; and we want an oncology/hematology center. That's why I'm still doing this. I want to help the community—whether it's to build a Rosenwald School [see page 132],[30,31] or get you to your appointment. This is the real world and this is a real life experience. I can either step away or step fully in and make sure the lack of access and inequity doesn't happen to another person ever again. I step in."

Chaplain Manager Dianne Horton's Roots

"My grandfather spent a lot of time in the hospital when I was young. I remember sitting in a waiting room and noticing this person coming around and speaking to people. I learned she was a chaplain. And as a little girl, I thought it was nice that she came around to just listen to people, to talk to them. Fast-forward to today: My dad lost a dear childhood friend of more than seventy years recently. The friend and his wife were in a terrible car wreck—she died first and then my dad's friend. My mom shared there was a large family gathering in the ICU during this stressful time and the chaplain had come by. She told me how touched they all were that this person came and listened to and prayed with them. That's the heart of this work for me, the privilege to be that person, to listen, to hold hands, to pray with people, to share some light and love. We meet people at the worst times in their lives with no judgment. We just do what we do—no matter who you are—and it helps."

CHAPLAIN MANAGER ADAM RIDENHOUR'S ROOTS

"I knew I wanted to go into ministry but my heart was with chaplaincy after a college internship with a chaplain. I knew I'd made the right choice when my eyes were further opened in a divinity school CPE class regarding the disparities around mental health. During school, I worked at the emergency department registration desk nights and weekends and would see the same people coming in week after week who were suicidal, homicidal, or needed a warm place to stay in the winter or a cool place to sit during the summer. So, that expanded my thinking and I went the counseling route. FaithHealth was the logical next step on my personal journey to address, from a trauma-informed care perspective, the disparities in our communities that lead to acute crises and more complex health concerns. Chaplain managers wear three hats, spiritual, mental, and social or population health, which represent three aspects and three different contracts with individuals. But they are alike in one important way—they are all about how we advocate for, accompany, walk beside, and speak with those on the fringes of our community. I love it more days than I don't."

Chaplain managers live in a world of dichotomies, a place that requires them to constantly and consistently straddle the pastoral and the procedural, ministry and management, heart and health. Sitting squarely in the Land of Both-And can feed the soul *and* try the patience. That's what makes the role so completely and unapologetically unique. Difficult. Rewarding.

Where chaplain managers live and work informs their day-to-day experience as much as the work itself, especially in smaller hospitals or rural communities. But no matter where they are or the size or type of population they serve, the principal goal of chaplain managers remains the same: to step into the breach and bridge the ever-widening chasm in care caused by the spiraling health and economic disparities that face the US population—especially the most vulnerable. According to the 2021 US Census, 19 percent of Americans had medical debt and could not afford to pay for their care in 2017.[32] A high medical debt burden was defined as representing more than 20 percent of the household's income—a significant and potentially catastrophic amount for approximately one in five Americans.[32] Data show that those most adversely affected by high medical debt are underserved and at-risk populations, people in fair to poor health, and individuals after a hospital stay or with a disability.[32] The average medical debt was $2000.[32]

Chaplain Managers Are Spiritual Care Professionals

As trained professional hospital chaplains, they meet patients, families, and hospital staff where they are by listening, praying, and holding the sacred space. They deliver unbiased, informed spiritual care in the healthcare setting to people of all faiths (or no faith) with no judgment and no agenda other than to help, whether it's providing crisis and grief support, connecting patients to community faith leaders, completing advance directives, or delivering counsel in times of spiritual distress or ethical dilemmas.[12]

WHO WE ARE: PEOPLE WHO STEP INTO THE GAP

Wilkes County is like a lot of rural communities in North Carolina: full of churches—mostly Baptist with a few Methodist, pentecostal, and Catholic. And as in many rural communities, chaplain managers are the people trained to go places traditional pastors may not be comfortable exploring. Case in point: suicide. When a young man in Graylin Carlton's community died by suicide and the pastor came to Carlton asking for professional support because he didn't know what to say to the family, Carlton sat down with them. He ended up doing the young man's eulogy. "We are here to meet people right where they are and give them the help they need in times of crisis, oftentimes right in the trenches of the community's culture gap."

Chaplain Managers Are Managers Within the Hospital System

While chaplain managers may feel like family to staff and patients, a big part of their job is management. They work within the infrastructure of the hospital to improve systems that may disrupt or negatively affect treatment. Because of their professional expertise, they serve on hospital teams ranging from diversity, equity, and inclusion, to crisis management, to budget discussions, to community health needs assessments, which annually document and seek to resolve important community health challenges. Thanks to their training and educational background, they support coworkers, administer Employee Emergency Fund monies, and sit in as an impartial observer and advocate during departmental disputes.

Chaplain Managers Are Community Organizers

In this era of value-based reimbursements, the drive to control costs by keeping patients out of the ED and a focus on outcomes founded on quality—instead of quantity—of care, true patient care doesn't start with a blood pressure cuff and end twenty minutes later with a prescription. The FaithHealth model is based on a 24/7/365 approach to health and well-being that includes helping patients get medical appointments *and* get *to* them, have access to health care *and* have a safe place to sleep, reduce barriers to health care *and* reduce hunger and food insecurity. The list is as diverse and unique as the nation's communities. That means chaplain managers spend a lot of time working *outside* the hospital on community coalitions, teams, committees, and boards. It's all about connections—connections to the hospital, connections to community resources, connections to faith organizations, and connections to the county and its people. Chaplain managers connect the dots, from hospital to patient to resources and back again, until people get the whole-person care they need.

Being a champion of community engagement is similar to the Christian story of Jesus feeding the five thousand. Chaplain managers always have a handful of loaves and a fish or two up their sleeves because of their roles in community committees, boards, advocacy groups, and initiatives. Many small and rural hospital settings don't have public transportation, a food bank, or a shelter for people experiencing homelessness. These small towns and agricultural areas can appear asset-deprived from a pure ethnographic perspective. But the FaithHealth lens empowers chaplain managers and their communities to rethink the way those assets look and shine a brighter light on them. Chaplain managers drive those narratives by being the creative thinkers who ask "what if ...?" Time and again, their answer to that question is often the same: What initially looks like a deficit may actually have some organic qualities that are really assets just waiting to be tapped—assets that are often left fallow due to a lack of connection or trust. Chaplain managers are trained to step into those gaps to take that fresh, hard look, and then, thanks to consistent and authentic relationship-building, turn deficits into determination—*and* action.

WHO WE ARE: A VOICE FOR THE VOICELESS

It's a given: Not everyone has a seat at the table. Chaplain managers have that seat and use it for advocacy. Being at the middle of the triangle between hospital and community can be an uncomfortable role. Because of their extensive training in trauma-informed care and their understanding of the need for safety, empowerment, and support, chaplain managers are committed to being present to hear both sides and speak up for those who don't have a seat. At an Opioid Settlement Fund meeting in Lexington County, Dianne Horton and a team of community advocates tried to persuade local politicians to channel some of the funds into housing and shelters. When told by one commissioner that more beds weren't needed because people who were unhoused had mental health issues and wouldn't follow the shelter rules, Horton swiftly pivoted and said, OK, let's speak to the mental health issues instead and how we can help out there. A big part of using the chaplain manager voice to guide the conversation and collective conscience is to speak truth to power—and walk the talk. "It's a privilege to have a seat at the table," she said. "It's our honor to hear and hold the stories, to be a voice for the voiceless, and inspire action and healing."

Chaplain Managers Are Advocates

One of the principle roles of chaplain managers is advocating for equitable treatment of all people, both inside and outside the walls of the hospital. They not only provide guidance on the hospital's Ethics Team and DEI Committee (Diversity, Equity, and

Inclusion) but, more importantly, they walk the talk on honoring patients' rights, aligning with their wishes, and supporting their autonomy. When families and the medical team are at odds on what "Do no harm" actually means to patients and what the most beneficial next steps might be, chaplain managers are invited to sit in on those consultations—not to share opinions, but to be a neutral (often, healing) presence in the room, empowered to facilitate conversation, advocate for the patient, and ensure respect for their autonomy. The real gift is simple—*and* powerful: to help both sides *really* hear each other. Families and patients often have difficulty grasping medical lingo. Because chaplain managers bridge the two worlds of the hospital and the community, they understand the jargon and can remind the medical team to communicate in the community's common language so it's understandable and accessible, or interpret the recommendations as needed. In a sense, chaplain managers are peace-makers and way-showers.

Chaplain Managers Are Cultural Brokers

While united in a mission to provide meaningful health care, The How of smaller hospitals in rural settings can be very different than in larger urban medical centers, especially during the uncertainty, and yes, grief that comes with mergers and the inevitable transition in personnel and services. It's vital that someone weaves the disparate elements of a community undergoing change—the new doctors and hospital staff—into the fabric of the community. It's an opportunity for understanding, creativity, connection, and often, peace-making. But it takes work. And with their expertise in navigating complicated and difficult emotional waters, that effort usually falls within the chaplain manager's scope, because they are the professionals with a foot in both worlds: the hospital and the community.

Chaplain managers fill the integral role of helping the community understand what the hospital team is doing and why. Equally important is helping physicians and specialists within the system understand the patients and the unique small-town culture they are serving—whether that culture is based on ethnicity, socioeconomics, nationality, history, or shared trauma. It's a type of healthcare map-making, with the chaplain managers helping medical professionals sensitively and compassionately navigate their community's unique demographics to, ultimately, build trust and meet the need. But it's quite the feat of social engineering, as chaplain managers are building the bridge out from *both* shores at the same time—from the hospital on one end and from the community on the other—hoping to meet solidly in the middle. Chaplain managers help build community.

WHO WE ARE: CULTURAL BROKERS
WILLING TO STEP INTO THE UNKNOWN

The COVID pandemic was a time that tested the mettle and tempered the steel of chaplain managers in their three primary roles: providers of pastoral care, members of the hospital management team, and trusted community partners. Adam Ridenhour delivered spiritual support to patients, families, and hospital staff impacted by coronavirus, including round-the-clock Code Lavender work to ease the stress of hospital peers afraid to go home to their children after being in a COVID patient's room all week. Code Lavender is an internal hospital protocol that supports stressed hospital staff during times of personal challenge. As a manager, he provided Code Lavender support following global events: assessed PPE needs (personal protective equipment, such as masks) and planned meaningful safety and disease prevention strategies. On the community side, he was part of extending hospital resources to community partners by sitting in on meetings about safe practices, setting up virus-related medical Q&As, and working with church volunteers who created an emergency shelter with cots for hospital staff concerned about going home and possibly exposing their families. When the hospital was gifted with an overabundance of PPE, he facilitated delivering them to the Baptist mission to distribute to vulnerable populations. "It wasn't enough to simply care for people during this frightening time; we were called to do and be more," Ridenhour said. "No matter the crisis, we are tasked with bringing hands and feet to spirituality, and to use our listening and counseling skills to support the health and well-being of our community—both inside and outside the hospital walls."

Based on these overarching ways of being as pastoral care providers, hospital managers, and community builders, the roles and responsibilities of chaplain managers in smaller hospitals or rural areas may include:

- Spiritual care: providing pastoral support for patients, families, and hospital staff
- Institutional chaplain functions within the hospital: training chaplain associates and connectors and leading or participating in prayer breakfasts, memorial services, team leaders meetings, etc.
- DEI Committee: serving on or leading the hospital's diversity, ethics, and inclusion team
- Workplace violence prevention: serving on or leading the hospital's team
- Code Lavender: leading the team that strategically and meaningfully supports stressed hospital staff undergoing personal challenges
- Mortality review: reading deceased patients' charts to assess hospital system failures and OFIs (opportunities for improvement)
- Daisy Committee: coordinating the hospital's nursing excellence award

- BEE Committee: leading the hospital's recognition of outstanding certified nursing assistants (CNAs)
- Hospital Foundation boards: serving on the team
- Employee Emergency Fund: managing the financial assistance program for hospital staff facing personal challenges
- Incident Command Team/Emergency Management Team: supporting the hospital's crisis intervention group and aiding in training efforts to help staff navigate weather events, shootings, bombings, catastrophic accidents, floods, etc.
- Safety coach: reviewing safety processes related to preventable hospital incidents involving patients
- BERT (Behavioral Escalation Response Team): de-escalating the troubling or dangerous behavior within the hospital of a patient, team member, or visitor
- Health Equity Pharmacy Program: supporting this initiative which provides psycho-social assistance to eliminate barriers to a patient receiving and correctly using medicines
- Family Reunification Team: working to reconnect patients and their families during disasters
- Bioethics Team: assessing and making recommendations if ethical concerns arise within the hospital
- CHNAs (Community Health Needs Assessment): as part of the hospital's justification for 501(c)(3) status, leading or working with the team that annually assesses community health challenges, and then working within the hospital and with outside organizations to create programs and projects that enhance well-being
- Community Benefits Team: similar to the CHNA process, assessing and making recommendations regarding the hospital's contribution to the community
- Caregiver Academy: setting up community lunch n' learns featuring local agency speakers to educate family caregivers on supporting patients

- Living wills, advanced directives, health care power of attorney: educating and supporting patients and the community
- Community nonprofits, advisory boards, grants committees, and leadership teams (United Way, homeless shelters, food banks): serving on or chairing teams
- Ministers groups: meeting with community pastors

While the responsibilities are as diverse as the chaplain manager's geographic area, county demographics, and community challenges, there is a common denominator of these seemingly discrete areas of service: The chaplain manager is firmly, sometimes uncomfortably, always necessarily, in the middle. On the one hand, the work is soul-satisfying; on the other hand, it can be heart-wrenching. It's not just a job, it's a calling. Not just a career, it's a journey, one the chaplain manager takes very seriously: walking each other home, hand-in-hand with the hospital and the community, with a destination of equal access to wholeness for all. But don't for one minute doubt that being a link in a long and twisted chain is easy. It's hard. But most days, it's a job to love.

> *"We are the liaison to the community, and that's a true benefit. Traffic goes both ways: We connect people to the hospital and the hospital to the community. If someone wants to know who to call within the medical system, we can help. We are the bridge."*
>
> — Dianne Horton

"It's hard when you are continually following a crisis client to the ED. But those issues that make you want to let go of the job are also the things that keep you in the work. It's the moments when we see breakthroughs in patients, when a church decides to open a transport ministry because they see a need in the community, when someone with vision faces an issue head-on by getting a grant to offer free counseling to farmers and farm workers—those are the prophetic pieces I want to be a part of."

— Adam Ridenhour

"We're needed because some people can't call anybody else for a ride to their hospital appointment because they live thirty-five miles away. We're there when they phone the hospital because they don't know who else to call and tell, 'I'm sitting in my house and it's snowing outside and I'm cold because I don't have heating oil.' And so, in a day and a time when people are siloing themselves, and this group of people believes this and the other group of people believe that, we're the ones who hold people's hands and meet them right where they are."

— Graylin Carlton

Who We Are: Dos and Don'ts

While it's easy to list the roles and responsibilities—The What of a job—it's much harder to figure out The How. Good thing chaplain managers are tasked with being creative, entrepreneurial, and dedicated. This list of Dos and Don'ts sharpens the blurry edges a little, giving shape and form to how to "show up" in the ever-evolving day-to-day activities.

DO prioritize. When faced with choosing between the most urgent or the loudest need, remember: Immediate and personal care are the most important. Focus on the crucial functions first, which naturally dovetails with the next three Dos ...

DO set and honor your boundaries. Boundary leadership requires rest and self-compassion.

DO work to have a good relationship with your leader—that support is vital, professionally and personally.

DO rely on your chaplain manager peers for feedback, insight, and support.

DON'T make hard and fast plans and then get frustrated when everything changes. Instead ...

DO be flexible and let the day unfold. Just move through it and make things happen, as you can.

DON'T try to juggle everything. Instead ...

DO what you can, not what you can't; roll with things and do the work as it comes.

DO take advantage of the freedom and creativity the role provides but...

DON'T take it personally when you hit a wall sometimes. It comes with the territory when you're balancing the procedural system of the hospital with the real-world demands of citizens in a community.

DO know your limitations. Accept that you can't be everything to everybody, which means ...

DON'T cringe or beat yourself up when you have to say "no, it's not my field of expertise."

4.

For the Good of the Hive:
Community Engagement

"Health doesn't just live inside the walls of the hospital."

— Adam Ridenhour

"A lot of this job is about being able to connect and build bridges with people."

— Dianne Horton

"We are the nexus of connection and care that helps to improve access to health and well-being. What that looks like is different in different counties."

— Emily Viverette

"It's part of our chemistry as chaplains to say 'OK, let's see what I can do to help.'"

— Graylin Carlton

Chaplain Managers: The Trusted Source (and Resource)

Nothing refined the silver of the healthcare system soul like the fire of the COVID-19 pandemic. At a time when science and medical recommendations were constantly—and rightly—evolving as new data was gathered, the hospital needed a trusted emissary to share the latest developments. Because of the relationships he had built in the community, as well as the trust of his hospital administration, Adam Ridenhour was perfectly positioned to move to the front lines and speak to local congregations in his communities, successfully brokering arrangements to have the hospital's chief medical officer present the real facts regarding the safety, prevention, and treatment recommendations—likely saving lives. "It's a trusted relationship, an extension of and a testament to how chaplains are respected across institutions in terms of holding confidentiality, doing what's right, ethical, moral, and good for patients," Ridenhour said. "Our hospital and community leaders have faith in us extending those same qualities, ways of being, and trusted relationships faithfully and thoughtfully to the entities we partner with. We aren't just another referral agency; we journey with the community we serve."

This is the quintessential chaplain manager in action—and the principal differentiator of this role from other chaplaincy models: community engagement. Equal parts minister and manager, community activist and cultural broker, chaplain managers, no matter which hat they are wearing, are trusted companions dedicated to accompanying their flock—whether a patient in the hospital or back home in the community—on whatever journey they are on in the moment.

A History of Community Engagement

> "FaithHealth reminds us, the fact is, in good conscience, you can't and should not separate the hospital from the community."
> — Emily Viverette

Where there is no vision, the people perish.[33] This proverb is as true today as it was in biblical times, as viable for healthcare systems and the communities they serve as it was for the ancient Jewish cultures of the Middle East. How you uncover and demonstrate a vision of care that people will get behind and, more importantly, live into is an integral part of today's healthcare evolution. Where does that transformation lead? Ask any chaplain manager and they will tell you the same thing: It leads to equal and just access to care for all.

How do you get there? For each chaplain manager the journey is as different as the healthcare system they work for and the community they serve. But the raison d'etre of all chaplain managers is the same: the certainty that health and well-being are inalienable human rights and that true health can only be achieved if it is accessible both within *and* outside the hospital walls. That's the guiding principle of the FaithHealth paradigm: Most of a patient's life happens in the community; therefore, that's where most health and healing should occur. FaithHealth is intentionally designed to be an innovative, dynamic partnership of faith groups, health systems, and communities focused on improving health. *That's* where the rubber hits the road, and why community engagement is a critical part of the role chaplain managers serve in their hospitals.

ENGAGEMENT AS UNIQUE AS THE COMMUNITY

Wilkes County's FaithHealth efforts have established a free transportation ministry to drive patients to medical appointments. In Lexington County, it's a partnership with a locally-owned grocery store to provide emergency food support to patients. In Davie County, FaithHealth shows up as part of a Healthy Farmers Initiative to deliver spiritual education, resources, counseling, and pastoral support to farmers experiencing isolation and despair. For every nonprofit in a community, every board, every new initiative, it's likely a chaplain manager has been invited to participate. "Being in all these meetings, it just happens—whether it's helping a lady with her transportation to the doctor or assisting the guy who just had a stroke and now is in a wheelchair and needs a ramp on his house or supporting the family with no funds to cremate a loved one who passed away at the hospital," Graylin Carlton said "You get to know the people who are doing the work, you connect with them, and you too become a resource for getting things done for people. I don't have to look for things to do. It just shows up every day. And every day I'm here to help."

Historically, community engagement has always been an important facet of North Carolina Baptist Hospital (now Atrium Health Wake Forest Baptist Hospital), the mother ship of North Carolina's FaithHealth model. When the hospital opened, it included a School of Nursing whose mission was to prepare nurses to serve in communities across the state. When the contractor, J.A. Jones, handed over the keys to the new eighty-eight bed hospital in Winston-Salem in May, 1923, he said "Well, here's the key, but there's not much need for it, since a hospital's door should never be locked to the sick."[34,35,36] It's the job of chaplain managers to ensure that unlocked door swings both ways—care should happen within the hospital *and* out in the community.

Proposed in 1919 at the annual Baptist State Convention just after the devastating worldwide flu pandemic, the hospital's purpose was loud and clear: to provide care, especially to those unable to pay. It was stated, "To those who are sick and need care the Baptist Hospital is the House of Healing. This institution is more than a building of red brick and mortar. Beneath its sturdy exterior beats the heart of humanity."[34,35,36] Chaplain managers exemplify that purpose, working to extend the institution and its heart of humanity outside the walls of the institution.

The fact that spiritual care was a key component of healing is what made the hospital unique. Rev. G.T. Lumpkin, the hospital's first superintendent (president), was a Baptist pastor who had served congregations in North Carolina and Virginia. Devoted to providing spiritual care to patients, their families, and staff, he laid the foundation of today's community engagement by also providing theological education to the nursing staff to prepare them for their work with local congregations.[34,35,36] That connection to congregations is still a key component of the system's spiritual care offerings. Today, chaplain managers create meaningful, collegial relationships with the local priests, rabbis, imams, and protestant ministers to ensure diverse spiritual resources are available to all patients and colleagues inside the hospital.

In the early days, community engagement was a two-way street. A Sewers and Stitchers club of Winston-Salem Baptist ministers' wives outfitted a large room at the Zinzendorf Hotel on Main Street with borrowed and rented sewing machines and made hundreds of linens for the hospital—from operating room and obstetrical linens to bed gowns and ward curtains.[34,35,36] The candles that lit the hospital hallways were donated by Moravians, a five-hundred-year-old Christian denomination originated in the Czech Republic and with a strong Winston-Salem community.[37] This boots-on-the-ground support of the hospital by congregations is still in action today. During the long, dark early days when COVID was at its most virulent and deadliest stages, chaplain managers reached out to faith communities for support. Congregations courageously opened up their buildings to provide havens for hospital staff to sleep when it didn't feel safe to go home to family. They also generously donated funds, food, and comfort bags to support those working on the frontlines in the hospital.

A Match Made in Heaven: Congregations and Community Engagement

The work of American community engagement has its roots in the Christian church of more than two centuries ago. According to the book *Christian Social Innovation*, diverse faith communities of the time of the Founding Fathers were part of the engine of innovation, growth, strength, and vitality: starting schools and colleges, opening hospitals and retirement facilities, building housing and food programs. Yet in recent decades, many Christian churches have taken a step back from social entrepreneurship.[38] Reconnecting those dots and reigniting that heart for community service is central to the FaithHealth model and the chaplain manager's work.

A COMMUNITY APPROACH TO HEALTH

Due to the high prevalence of strokes and heart attacks in the Black community, Graylin Carlton paved the way for the Wilkes Medical Center's heart unit to meet with the only Black Presbyterian church in the county about a Q&A to raise awareness about AFib, its warning signs and impacts. The church hosted a hospital clinician who answered questions from the large crowd, which included congregants from every Baptist church in the county. "That blew my mind," Carlton said. "It's a rare thing to get that kind of church crossover. It turned out just wonderfully. This event helped build trust many ways—in the community, between the church denominations, and at the hospital. Our hospital was on shaky ground here with the African-American community because of the past. This really built some bridges in Wilkes County."

It's part of the job of chaplain managers to know if a patient needs food, legal help, housing, clothing, or transportation—and then to act on that knowledge with meaningful support and access to resources. That's the real-world reason why connections outside the hospital walls are so important. The truth is, the way the FaithHealth model sees it, there is no wall. And the logical choice is to team up with faith communities, as well as service organizations. But going "outside the walls" is more than just partnering with local clergy to deliver spiritually-appropriate care to constituents inside the hospital. It is active community engagement to impact population health, per the mission and mandate of the hospital.

CONGREGATIONS + MEDICAL CENTERS = COMMUNITY CARE

Similar to clinicians, chaplain managers have caseloads of patients they work with to lower barriers to care and enhance well-being. They follow their patients along the healing journey to ensure access to a number of key supports of good health: food, housing, transportation, education, and a primary care physician and medicines. Chaplain managers recruit congregations to be a part of the popular MedAssist program, a statewide North Carolina nonprofit pharmacy which distributes free prescription and over-the-counter medicines to neighbors in need. Nonprofits participate by setting up booths and sharing information on resources they can provide in times of trouble. "This is a big deal in our county and a really good tool for bringing people together," said Graylin Carlton. "It helps people get the medicines they need, it helps the hospital in its mission to ensure the health of the community, and it helps nonprofits and agencies get their message out and do more good. Plus, we talk with each other—chaplain managers, clergy, medical teams, and nonprofit staff. We exchange business cards and ideas. We build bridges to help each other and the community."

But sometimes, the task of community engagement with faith communities can be challenging. Partnerships are as variable and unique as the people in them and the cultures, dogmas, and belief systems that guide them. Chaplain managers are trained to step into that space of discomfort, confusion, and misunderstanding that surrounds certain issues, such as suicide, addiction, and end-of-life decisions, that faith communities can't, won't, or don't know how to engage with in a way that comforts, lifts up, and heals. The chaplain manager can be that rock-solid bridge in the middle, uniting the two sides—the person needing support and their church leaders—in understanding and compassion.

> ### Faith Communities and Hospitals: A Partnership That Works
>
> A pastor came to Dianne Horton about hosting a traditionally difficult conversation in his predominantly Black community: advanced directives regarding end-of-life medical care in the hospital. The hospital provided the education at the Black church host site. The panel discussion of experts included a medical provider, attorney, pastor, and funeral home director, as well as documents for attendees to complete, as needed. The hospital relied on the trust and goodwill built by the church and its community to encourage attendance—and it worked. The event was well-received at the packed house of worship, and served as a stepping stone to strong partnership in future community crises, including the COVID pandemic. "It was important that the church sponsored this and not the hospital," said Horton. "People trust their pastor and their friends at church. That partnership was what got people in the door to hear the education. That partnership increased the community's trust in me and my work. The same event held at the hospital would not have had nearly the same attendance. That's the job of a chaplain manager: looking at a community and a situation and deciding the best way to meet people where they are spiritually, mentally, emotionally, and physically."

While many faith communities may no longer have the resources to launch a school or build a nursing home, they *can* come alongside a mission such as FaithHealth. They *can* participate in

Wilkes Medical Center's Adopt-a-Unit program, supplying snacks for dedicated health care staff. They *can* provide goodie bags of personal hygiene products (toothbrushes, paste, lotion, etc.) for Winston-Salem campus nurses to give to patients in need. They *can* assemble care bags of products and treats with inspirational messages and thank-you notes for Lexington's staff during crises, such as COVID. They *can* donate to Ebenezer's Attic in Wilkes County, a free clothing closet that underserved patients can shop for underwear, socks, shirts, and shoes. They *can* host a MedAssist event so that neighbors don't have to choose between buying food and buying medicine. And FaithHealth comes alongside congregations' missions to love one another in the form of transportation programs that take people to grocery stores and the pharmacy and by sharing COVID resources, such as masks and accurate information about vaccines and best practices.

The invitation is the same today as it was hundreds of years ago: tap into the hunger of faith communities to stay relevant and encourage them to get involved. The FaithHealth lens laser-sharpens that focus to a single mission: How to really partner with a community to examine and resolve how society is missing the mark on access to the hospital and healing? In rural communities that missed mark is day-to-day physical access.

What Community Engagement Looks Like Day to Day

> *"If we are spiritual care advocates, as well as advocates of social engagement and behavioral health, we must remember that health doesn't just live inside the medical center—it's about health in the community too."*
>
> — Adam Ridenhour

> *"You have to be able to, on the fly and in the moment, see all the angles. If you're dealing with a domestic violence situation, that means you have to also look at the possibility of an unhoused situation, food insecurity, and mental health effects. Everything ties together."*
>
> — Graylin Carlton

Population health is as much getting to know people and standing in the trenches with them in times of trouble as it is performing an operation and writing a prescription. More and more, hospitals are discovering that building strong community connections positively impacts population health—physical, behavioral, social, and mental health. Ensuring there is a legacy of care that follows patients once they leave the hospital and reenter their community is vital. Yes, community engagement is a formalized part of the chaplain manager job description, but it is also a spiritual calling. While a hospital administrator can ask the chaplain manager to establish a relationship with a new nonprofit or attend a community meeting to connect with an organization's executive director, there is also autonomy in decision-making, permission to get creative, and the freedom to move quickly. It's the perfect union of plan and action, faith and works: following a mandate *and* following up on transportation for a patient who needs a ride to the doctor.

The symbiosis between hospitals and communities is The New Normal in the value-based health care world, with the added benefit of bringing a chaplaincy lens to societal problems and social justice issues. Chaplain managers are expert at finding a vacuum and discovering creative ways to address it. They provide the topography of the hospital's map of population health by operationalizing an implementation plan and telling the qualitative stories of the community to accompany the data. Their role of community engagement is to bridge the disconnect between data analytics and on-the-ground care. It's one thing to show diversity, equity, and inclusion statistics; it's another thing entirely to share stories of how these efforts have impacted a community longitudinally. Yes, you can show data, but hearing the real-world implications on real people is profound. That's the FaithHealth model—to combine the metrics on outreach efforts with the stories on impacting lives. Whether it's listening empathetically, bringing on-board faith communities, or spotlighting a place of justice, chaplain managers breathe life into the necessary spreadsheets and flow charts.

> *"We bring that justice. While population health does the research and delivers the statistics, we implement it, we make it happen because of the trust we've built being in the community. We see it on paper, but when the rubber meets the road, we're the ones doing it, we're the ones implementing the plans on paper. A lot of times in small hospitals and rural communities, there's a lot of paperwork but things don't always happen. We develop relationships, we bring together people who are never together, we make it happen."*
> — Graylin Carlton

Chaplain managers spend between a third and half of their time on community engagement, most of it in conversation around the community table—often with the same individuals, always with the same goal: to help people heal in every way. The community tables where Graylin Carlton, Dianne Horton, and Adam Ridenhour sit include the local United Way board, Family Promise (an organization that seeks to end homelessness), the hospital's workplace violence committee, the community domestic violence task force, the county's opioid prevention team, a Rosenwald school board, the chamber of commerce board, their medical center's Health Foundation Board and committees, hospice, family services, a prison reentry program, a homelessness recovery care system, Caregiver Academy (a speakers series designed to educate caregivers), their local ministerial associations, senior services, the aging committee, and the local mental health collaborative.

"There comes a point where we need to stop just pulling people out of the river. We need to go upstream and find out why they're falling in."
— Desmond Tutu

Access to Care: A Guiding Mandate

While today it's easy to call a ride service like Uber, that wasn't the case in rural Wilkes County a few years ago. One of the county's main challenges was access to medical care—literally: for patients without a vehicle to physically get to their medical appointments. Transportation was a real barrier to care. Graylin Carlton led the charge in breaking through that barrier: from designing a program and getting grant funding, to identifying and connecting with an agency to provide transportation and answering the phone. "This was a big deal, making all the connections to help patients in Wilkes County get the care they need at home, outside the walls of the hospital," he said. "Our job as community chaplain is to make sure we communicate with the health department, the pastors, and the local ministries and nonprofits to make things happen. It's important that we hear the heartbeat of the community and have these kinds of partners to work with." Davie County's Adam Ridenhour is quick to point out that initiatives such as Carlton's transportation program have enormous impact on the community. "We are able to put together the puzzle pieces between campuses, clinics, and organizations, along with the grant monies to support it. Because of our role, we can broker resources and match them up to people who need them that others in the hospital system might not be able to."

> "Our job is to look for the voices in the community. We all know the loud voices, that person who is the mover and shaker. But we also need to keep our eyes and ears open for the quiet strength of a person who is working behind-the-scenes to make things happen. In our community, one man was behind almost every nonprofit and good idea, so if we followed his lead, it would open doors."
> — Dianne Horton

Bringing Accountability to Access: The Community Health Needs Assessment (CHNA)

> "Having a chaplain manager puts a good face on the hospital, having a person who actually goes into the community to help patients versus them having to come to us as usual. It shows investment in the community."
> — Dianne Horton

> "Our job as community chaplains and with CHNAs is to make sure we communicate with the health department, the pastors, and the local ministries to make things happen. It's important that we hear the heartbeat of the community and have these kinds of partners to work with."
> — Graylin Carlton

One of the centerpieces of the work of population health in nonprofit hospitals is the Community Health Needs Assessment (CHNA). The CHNA is a crucial part of the hospital's justification for 501(c)(3) status and is part of the reporting for the Affordable Care Act (ACA).[7,11] Conducted every three years, this summary of county health services data helps shape the hospital's commitment to serve the broader health of the community, especially in the arenas of disparity and health equity, and informs how the hospital allots their community benefit—its programs that serve the community.[8,12]

Chaplain managers lead or are a part of the team that annually assesses community health challenges for the CHNA. They analyze the CHNA results and make recommendations regarding the hospital's contribution to the community. Then, they work within the hospital and with outside organizations to strategically align resources and create an implementation plan of initiatives and projects to meet the identified needs and enhance community health and well-being. They often also write the final community benefit report, which include metrics for assessing those benefits.

The transportation program in Wilkes County was a direct result of a CHNA report, which was the primary tool for writing and winning a grant to fund the initiative to break through the barrier to access to care and get patients without a vehicle to their medical appointments. It was a CHNA report that revealed the need to support the mental and spiritual health of area farmers. The CHNA inspired collaboration with Davie County's The Bridge, a one-stop shop for services in the rural, economically-challenged town of Cooleemee. This church-run program offered a medical transportation ministry, weekly meals, resources for job-hunting, counseling, housing, and a mobile food pantry. Chaplain managers often function as grant-writers, fundraisers, steering committee members, and chief bottle-washers to support the new projects—whether it's a community transportation program or a hospital improvement project.

MEETING THE NEED AT THE MOMENT OF THE NEED

When Adam Ridenhour first started as a chaplain manager, he had a Connector (a part-time, lightly funded role of providing hands-on care in the community, such as delivering meals, and recruiting and training volunteers) who was happy to drive patients wherever they needed to go. But as hospital contracts changed, that service changed. The Connector could no longer serve that vital function ... which created a void that needed to be filled. A group formed, assessed the problem, traveled to investigate other communities' solutions, and is currently implementing its own transportation program. "There is no way I wanted to jump into transportation issues—it's not my training or interest," said Ridenhour, whose expertise centers on mental health and counseling. "But when the needs are loud enough, you address what must be addressed and you start to see the interconnectedness of all those access points that call attention to what has to be done at the time. How we address a need is different for each of us, because our communities are unique. But it is clear that we can't simply turn away and say 'It's not a problem,' regardless of whether or not we have the support to try to find a solution. It's always a work-in-progress."

Why It's Not Social Work

"Most of the social workers are calling us for help, because of our placement in the community and knowing so many people and organizations beyond the resources they have on their list. But it's not just a list of resources—it's the people we know and can call on, because we have that relationship and work with them."
— Graylin Carlton

"Because of our job and skill set, we can say, OK, let's look at it this way. Chaplain managers are skilled at looking for the open window after the door has slammed shut."
— Emily Viverette

Social workers and case managers in health systems are charged with making sure patients have a safe discharge plan, which includes addressing basic needs so that patients are less likely to need another hospitalization in the near future. This is very similar to the community engagement role chaplain managers are tasked to do. The difference is the spiritual aspect chaplain managers bring to the job—and the freedom they're given to step in and support outside the walls. Chaplain managers seek to augment care and not duplicate the efforts of social work and case management.

Social workers must adhere to definitive guidelines and rules, with more implied and tangible terms and liabilities, and are often limited to working within the walls of the hospital and the parameters of resources known and available in a community. Chaplain managers often have broader relationships and connections because of their community engagement. They can share their contacts list for new initiatives that can help, connect social workers directly to the right person, and identify churches and other organizations that may be able to offer support.

It's a constant give and take. Chaplain managers connect the dots, they are the face of the hospital in the community and the bridge between the two. But don't be mistaken, that bridge travels both ways. The very same community agencies and resources the chaplain managers often refer patients and families to will ask questions and make suggestions about services at the hospital.

> *"Fortunately, our hospital care coordinators and social workers know lots of resources. What differentiates chaplain managers is being in on some of the community initiatives outside the hospital that lift up some of the grassroots efforts and supportive structures that may not be found in a web search or on a resource list. The role of chaplain manager provides flexibility to be in both places at once—in the hospital and out in the community."*
> — Adam Ridenhour

> "I find that I'm in a number of different community meetings but the same people are always at the table and we have bonded. So, we stay in communication. If I can't think of something or someone to help, I know who to call, I know where to go, I know how to connect."
> — Dianne Horton

Stone Soup

> "In rural hospitals, you realize pretty fast that The Man [boss] is not quite as important as the pastor of the corner church."
> — Graylin Carlton

> "You have to be able to plug into the hive mind."
> — Emily Viverette

We've all heard the story. Wayfarers carrying nothing but a large cauldron enter a small village and ask for food. It is hard times in the land, so they are turned down flat by the suspicious citizens. So they go to a river and fill their big pot with water, drop a river rock into it, and set it over a fire, stirring and sniffing at it appreciatively. Pretty soon, a villager walks up and asks about the steaming pot. The travelers tell him it is a tasty stone soup that they are happy to share, but it needs just a tad more flavor. The villager runs home and returns with a few carrots for the pot. Soon he is followed by a woman with a couple of potatoes. A family stops by with a large cabbage. A young farmer brings over a chicken. A little girl offers an onion. An elderly man has a little salt he can spare. On and on it goes until the whole village, chatting and laughing together, watches as, at last, the stone is pulled from the soup and set aside and everyone gets a bowlful of the delicious and nourishing meal.[39,40] But it is more than the body that is nourished—it is the spirit, it is the community, it is hope. When we share our resources with others, we all benefit. As we give, so we receive. A community that works to include everyone finds, well, unity. Understanding, acceptance, inclusion, and access heal communities.

Bottom line, chaplain managers don't work just for the hospital; they work for the good of the hive. They answer the invitation and *are* the change they want to see in the world. Like the wayfarers in the story, they help others recognize and use their gifts and resources to build strong community connections. In the chaplain manager world, those connections and that sense of community is a way to impact population health and help people feel whole. Just as water slowly but surely, inexorably and completely, finds its way into every nook and cranny, crevice and crack, the reach of chaplain managers, by design, is subtle yet everywhere. Their impact, by intention, is quiet yet profound. That's how community engagement works best.

> *"The majority of people's lives are spent outside the hospital, unless there's an emergency or a decline in health. Maintaining health and wholeness outside of the hospital is critical. That's what FaithHealth is really all about. Of course, a key aspect of wholeness is access."*
> — Dianne Horton

> *"Chaplains advocate for patients and the community, raising issues about access to care, the lack of mental health care and dental health care in certain settings. They examine and shine a light on how care is divided by socioeconomic status, gender issues, racial division, and more. Chaplain managers are charged with—called to—challenge systems of injustice, systems that promote divisions in communities—both outside and inside the hospital walls."*
> — Adam Ridenhour

5.

Nailing Jello to the Wall:
Measuring the Impact of Chaplain Managers

"Not everything that counts can be measured and not everything that can be measured counts."

— Albert Einstein

This is going to be a short chapter. The reason? Because proving bottom line impact in the spiritual care world is like nailing Jello to the wall. It's impossible to make it stick. How can you financially quantify trust, a shoulder to lean on, and peace of mind? What price do you set for deep listening skills and cultural humility? Where on a spreadsheet is the asset entry for chaplaincy? It can be especially hard to assess in the health care industry, where every service, every product, every procedure, and every interaction is rigorously coded and billed, and costs are constantly under scrutiny. Just like doctors and nurses, aides and physical therapists, x-ray technicians and anesthesiologists, chaplain managers are hands-on providers of care. They are the strong links in an often complex chain connecting the local hospital with the community and the community with the local hospital. And yet the results chaplain managers achieve are more ephemeral and harder to pin down. In the moment, the resources and access, peace and sanctuary, they provide to patients, teammates, and their communities, the compassionate yet savvy ability to build on the strengths and spiritual assets of the people they serve, are priceless. And that's the problem: It's price-less.

Despite a number of small studies showing that chaplain care is associated with higher levels of patient and family satisfaction with hospital care, there are no large-scale, evidence-based, rigorously-designed metrics on the benefit of chaplains in the health care setting.[41] The question is complex. While the case can be made anecdotally for chaplain care at end-of-life and hospice stages, there is no statistical proof that spiritual support for *all* patients is a plus for a hospital.[41] Then, why does Atrium Health Wake Forest Baptist, a large and renowned academic health system with a children's hospital, five community hospitals, over three hundred primary and specialty clinics, twenty-seven hundred physicians, and a prestigious associated medical school, put so much emphasis on the chaplain manager model in its rural hospitals? Who decided to promote these chaplains to managers, assigned to important hospital teams and committees, including DEI (Diversity, Equity, and Inclusion), Employee Emergency Fund, and disaster/crisis teams? Who invited them to sit in on interdepartmental disputes? Why do chaplain managers stay so connected to their hospital leaders? How do they become respected community movers and shakers outside the walls of the hospital? While it's hard to pinpoint, obviously someone is doing something right. There is a growing recognized value in health care for the entrepreneurial efforts and change agency of chaplain managers—especially in small and rural hospitals and communities. But *proving* it? That's harder.

Researchers agree: More study is needed to heighten awareness of the pivotal contributions chaplains make to patients' health care experiences and to promote deeper interdisciplinary understanding and relationships within the hospital.[42] But how to achieve real-world results? FaithHealth's unique model—getting patients to the right door at the right time, ready to be treated and never alone—*can* affect the bottom line. This initiative, a partnership between health care systems, congregations, and community agencies and advocacy organizations, is designed to save the hospital and patients money, especially the higher costs of delayed treatment for medical conditions-turned-crises. FaithHealth supports the marginalized by increasing their access to care, improves community health, and ultimately saves lives. It's a tall enough order to forge a new trail, much less create a system to measure impact. The role of chaplain manager, the people positioned inside hospitals to help activate the FaithHealth mission, is still young—at work in North Carolina only since 2012.

Making patients partners in their health care makes sense for hospitals—*dollars and cents*. But that can be a challenge in smaller hospitals with fewer than one hundred beds. On the one hand, by their very nature, local hospitals have to rely more heavily on area faith communities and other agency and nonprofit resources to support patients who fall between the cracks. On the other hand, they often do not have chaplain managers (or chaplains, for that matter) on staff—the professionals trained in leveraging the very resources these smaller institutions and their patients need.[12]

In her thesis, *Building Bridges: Integrating Community Engagement Skills into Clinical Pastoral Education at Atrium Health Wake Forest Baptist*, Emily Viverette makes the case for the value of chaplain managers to small and rural hospitals. In this evolving era of health care reform, launched by the signing into law of the ACA in 2010 (Patient Protection and Affordable Care Act), increasing access to affordable health insurance (*and* care), expanding Medicaid coverage, and reducing costs through health care innovations can't happen in a vacuum.[12] Complicated by the demands of the current do-more-with-less world of higher costs and co-pays and lower insurance reimbursements, small and rural medical centers especially need innovative and engaged support in meeting the ACA goals. Add to that the profound business (and cultural) paradigm shift in the health care arena: from fee-for-service reimbursement to pay-for-value, from prioritizing emergent and acute care to focusing on prevention and wellness.[12] Enter the chaplain manager, a board-certified expert trained to help hospitals be good neighbors—especially to the underserved—and charged with actioning the Promethean ideals of the ACA: community, cooperation, communication, and collaboration[12]—the same ideals FaithHealth embraces ... ideals and activities that can be as hard to quantify as faith, as difficult to measure as love.

Providing spiritual care and building bridges in rural communities can be difficult because poverty, health and social disparities, racial injustice, divisiveness, and polarization—and the suffering and isolation that go with them—continue to be a challenge.[43] Still, those ACA ideals are the core strengths of small and rural communities. Viverette points out that social capital is crucial for hospitals in these locales. While they lag behind in almost every health care indicator compared to larger medical centers, rural hospitals excel in community connections and engagement.[12] Chaplain managers, often working in small or rural communities they know well, are skilled at identifying and leveraging those informal (and invaluable) networks for care that extend beyond the walls of the hospital after inpatient care has ended.

Chaplain Managers Leverage the Innate Strengths of Small Hospitals

As the number of rural hospitals and health care dollars shrink, making access to care even harder and removing a vital economic engine from their communities, the case can be made for having a board-certified spiritual care expert trained in community engagement and advocacy. One hundred thirty-six rural hospitals across the US closed from 2010 to 2021, with thirty-seven closing just since 2020, and six hundred more—approximately 30 percent of all rural hospitals in the US—at risk of closure.[6,7] Equal parts minister and advocate, activist and detective, interpreter and bridge-builder, community organizer and hospital manager, chaplain managers serve a decisive role in rural communities, on par with community health workers and behavioral health specialists. There are some significant rubber-meets-the-road benefits to having a chaplain manager on board at small or rural hospitals.

Taking on the Hard Jobs

By their very nature, background, and training, chaplain managers bring a unique perspective and voice to the teams they lead and participate in within the hospital. However, it's often the hard hospital teams they are required to engage with, the ones that require extra time, emotional intelligence, creativity—*and* work: DEI (Diversity, Equality, and Inclusion), Crisis, Ethics, Code Lavender, and the Employee Emergency Fund. Because flexibility, freedom, and entrepreneurship are required skills, and trust and confidentiality are a given, chaplain managers often take on—and accomplish—tasks other staff aren't available for.

Where There's a Will, There's a Way

Perhaps the chaplain manager's greatest skill is willingness. It's the ability to step into the unknown, to compassionately listen for the needs, to give a voice to the voiceless, and to tease out the possibilities. But it's something more. As Dr. Martin Luther King, Jr., pointed out, it's the faith to take the next step even when you can't see the whole staircase. Chaplain managers excel at taking that next step ... and the next one. Graylin Carlton's administrator invited him to represent the hospital on the Health Equity team because he knew Carlton was already at work addressing health equity issues in the community. "He wanted my good input on that," Carlton said. "My leader recognizes that we wear multiple hats, he sees the strengths we have, he knows we're familiar with the community, and he uses that to improve the hospital." Adam Ridenhour agrees that chaplain managers are masters of juggling multiple roles and seamlessly moving between worlds both inside and outside the hospital. Beyond the expected roles of spiritual care and accompaniment, chaplain managers are generalists: They are one of few in the hospital who serve multiple functions in multiple spaces, with the specificity to listen to the concerns of patients and teammates. Yet they are specialists with an impressively broad scope: They can serve on the hospital Workplace Violence Committee and their county's Aging Committee at the same time. "I think there's a big value in having someone like us on the team," Ridenhour said. "We not only fill the gaps between social support structures for patients in the community such as transportation but we also help hold various roles within a health system together too."

Ensuring a More Peaceful and Productive Workplace

Chaplain managers are invaluable aids in improving staff morale, retention, and productivity, which helps reduce the spiraling cost of turnover and the training of new hires. Because they are credentialed spiritual care specialists, chaplain managers provide a confidential shoulder for staff to lean on in times of trouble. Because they are trained listeners, hospital leadership will often invite them to sit in on departmental disputes to provide a safe space for sharing and to assess dynamics. Because they are managers, they oversee key hospital teams that directly impact staff well-being (DEI, Ethics, and Crisis), administer the hospital's Employee Emergency Fund, and lead the highly-valued Code Lavender program, which cares for stressed hospital staff undergoing personal challenges and was a lifesaver during the COVID pandemic. Because they are community organizers, they connect staff facing financial challenges to housing, food, and other support in times of need.

Supporting Staff, Generating Trust

Community engagement doesn't just happen outside the walls of the hospital. There is the strong—and traditional—call to first serve the community inside the hospital. Chaplain managers provide invaluable support to hospital teammates during times of crisis. When a staff member came to Dianne Horton for financial assistance, Horton went beyond putting in an application for Employee Emergency Funds, a program she managed. She also sat down with the team member to work up a budget. No matter what they did, there was no way the colleague could catch up financially, much less get ahead—the paycheck just wouldn't stretch that far. That was a hard reality for the staff member, affecting not only job performance but also mental health, physical health, family dynamics, and housing. So, Horton did what chaplain managers do: Because of her extensive network outside the hospital, she connected the employee to vital community resources that could help with housing, food, and transportation. "This story demonstrates the confidence that our teammates place in us, that they would bring their financial burden to me and lay it out," Horton said. "It's because we're chaplains. It's a sacred trust."

Walking the Talk:
The Community Health Needs Assessment (CHNA)

Atrium Health Wake Forest Baptist provided community benefit valued at $767.5 million in 2022; $15.4 million of it was designated for community health programs, operations, and donations, including FaithHealth initiatives, community health access, direct patient assistance, and other services.[44] The lynch pin of that vital contribution is the CHNA, Community Health Needs Assessment. Chaplain managers help create this document to ensure their nonprofit hospital is walking the talk of community engagement and benefit.

Chaplain managers and others in the hospital collaborate with the county health department and other health and well-being entities in the community to identify broad categories of challenges: access to care, substance abuse, misuse of medications, child and maternal health, and more. Once approved and funded by the hospital board, the final results of the CHNA can lead to real change in communities. The hospital sees the need, agrees with the value of solving the problem, and may invest in the opportunity to make a substantive difference. But beyond funding, the medical center leaves a large portion of program creation and implementation to the chaplain managers and their local partners. Data analyzed from the CHNA made it possible for Davie County to partner with a lung bus mobile screening program to serve local residents. It was the catalyst for writing the grant to fund a free transportation program for patients in Wilkes County. The CHNA also led to outreach initiatives in Davidson County with a local elementary school near the hospital. Food banks, shelters for people experiencing homelessness, rent assistance, opioid abuse interventions, and more are all ways that chaplain managers and their partners turned CHNA data into real access and support for the underserved in their communities. While the hospital may not always fund the programs and chaplain managers may not always write the grants, the chaplain managers are usually part of the team that's figuring out what's needed and how to activate the solution.

Addressing Social Drivers of Health

Respected and well-integrated into their interdisciplinary hospital teams, chaplain managers work with social workers and care coordinators to find resources for patients who fall through the cracks. Because it's a part of their job to be plugged into community teams and agencies, they are adept at skillful problem-solving and filling gaps. Patients with food, transportation, shelter, and hope are more likely to comply with medical instructions, prescriptions, and appointments, which means they are more likely to heal and not return to the hospital, which serves the new paradigm of value-based health care.

Proving Value through Change

One of the biggest problems small hospitals face is long wait times and back-ups in the emergency department (ED). Wilkes Medical Center Chaplain Manager Graylin Carlton was a key participant in a hospital Institutional Culture and Awareness Project to address the issue. Instead of adding more health care professionals to handle the crowd (the obvious fix), the improvement project team instead created new measures and improved systems to help patients more easily get to their doctors' appointments and receive their medications. The new process effectively eased the bottleneck in the ED and changed the busy department's workflow from everyday health care to true emergencies, demonstrating real impact on patient care and outcomes. These improvement programs—within and outside the hospital and funded by the medical center or outside grants—are often helmed by chaplain managers, who maintain close community contacts and keep an eagle eye on barriers to access and care. Other programs may include providing patients with support for utilities, groceries, rent, and transportation, which helps prevent homelessness and enhance overall health and well-being. A cold, hungry patient with no housing or transportation can't heal. "It's important to be part of the community process, but it's also important to remind the hospital what we committed to," Carlton said. "Our administration has made a commitment to the community and we can't just do lip service. Something has to be **done**. Chaplain managers help in that process."

Healing Communities

Chaplaincy is currency—and the revenue on that investment in compassion and fairness is goodwill, peace of mind, and trust. Chaplain managers are pivotal to healing communities—whether it's acknowledging and addressing a long history of mistrust due to racial tensions (the eugenics program, the Tuskegee experiments, etc.) or helping people navigate the more recent COVID pandemic, with its swiftly evolving strains, rapidly changing science, and politicization of containment efforts. Chaplain managers listen to their communities (both within and outside the hospital), help create programs, meet needs, and demonstrate reliability, transparency, and accountability, which are especially important in communities where trust has been broken.

Saving Money

Because they are generalists, chaplain managers wear a lot of hats and serve several functions in multiple spaces within the hospital universe: chaplain, counselor, community health worker, grant-writer, fundraiser, hospital manager, advocate, team leader, researcher, hospital representative on community boards, and community representative on hospital teams. The job description is as endless and organic as the hospitals and communities they support—whether it's serving as a community health worker arranging transportation for a patient who lives alone and needs a ride to a doctor's appointment, acting as a prayer partner with a hospital patient who is having a dark night of the soul moment, or joining in as a board member of the county's domestic violence committee. Other cost savings include being on the front-end of the team that keeps patients out of the ED by ensuring patients have a medical home and access to regular appointments. The bottom line is, well, the bottom line: Chaplain managers save the hospital money on staffing, and are one of the institution's greatest investments in the local community.

Creating Positive Buzz

Chaplain managers are the cheapest and best marketing a hospital could have because they are one of the primary public faces of the hospital in the community, making them significant and positive contributors to their center's reputation. There is great PR value in sitting on community teams, writing grants for new initiatives, and implementing life-changing programs that solve real-world problems.

PICKING UP THE PIECES

The time when chaplain managers shine brightest is during a crisis, helping pick up the pieces after a seminal event—whether it is the momentary compassionate support of family members after a patient's death or the 24/7 long-term support of teammates navigating the life-changing trauma of working in the hospital during COVID. Because they are chaplains, they are trained in compassionate response. Because they are managers, they can bring about change.

Supporting High-impact Care

Yet many of the hands-on initiatives chaplain managers help communities create to address barriers to access and social drivers of health *do* have measurable objectives and goals, delivering direct impact and outcomes and affecting lives and improving care. Wilkes County's transportation ministry partnership with SURGE, Lexington Medical Center's partnership with a locally-owned grocery store to provide emergency food support, and the Healthy Farmers program to deliver spiritual education, resources, counseling, and pastoral support to farmers experiencing isolation and despair are all community programs that can be measured and documented. Healthy Farmers is part of CareNet, a North Carolina network of state-licensed therapists providing community-based, personalized counseling services to individuals, families, and groups. Chaplain Manager Adam Ridenhour is a licensed CareNet counselor.

TRANSPORTATION PROGRAM PROVEN
TO REMOVE BARRIERS TO ACCESS

The Wilkes County transportation ministry created and managed by Chaplain Manager Graylin Carlton has had an enormous impact on care outcomes for county patients. Supported entirely by grants and with no hospital funding, the goals of this program were to reduce the likelihood that patients would cancel or be no-shows to their medical follow-up care appointments, increase the continuity of care for patient services, and help patients continue to receive care in their local communities. It is important to note that this ministry is not limited to transporting patients to only Atrium Health Wake Forest Baptist facilities. Over a two-year period (May, 2021, to May, 2023), the ministry provided patients with 1222 rides to health care providers, including sixty-two wheelchair assists, and forty-two holiday or weekend rides, at a cost of $159,061. In that twenty-four month period, there were only thirty-two no-shows, a phenomenally low 2.6 percent and a tribute to the excellent customer service and personal bonds that were formed. During that time, most of the trips were for dialysis (29 percent), followed by trips to the local or main hospital (21 percent). The average ride cost was $107 (the county is one hundred miles in length). "One of our main issues that we have grappled with was for patients in our rural communities to have access to health care," Carlton said. "There's no ride share service (e.g., Uber, cab service, Lyft, etc.) in Wilkes County and that was a big deal. So we created the transportation program. Making that connection has really helped the patients in our county get the care they need once they leave the hospital."

Proving Value Is All About Asking the Right Question

In a perfect world, chaplaincy would be so foundational to the hospital's success that its assigned CPT (current procedural terminology) codes would be activated for reimbursement and not limited to traditional spiritual care—a recognition that spiritual care was so pivotal to healing that it was covered by insurance companies. This goal is closer to reality today: There is an effort currently underway to utilize CPT codes for spiritual care services in some US hospital systems. In small hospitals and rural communities, chaplain managers represent a substantial investment—

but it's an investment in community-building (and sometimes, community preservation). In the relatively young value-based health care paradigm that is still struggling to find quantitative data to justify its own existence, asking chaplain managers, also in their relative infancy as a professional field, to do the same is like relying on AI (artificial intelligence) to write this book. It's too much too soon. For now. Plus, the field of population health is facing an identity crisis: trying to unite the data side with the human side, the metrics with community engagement. That wide disconnect between data analytics and on-the-ground care for the community affects how a hospital tells its story. Value-based health care can speak to the analytical aspect, but how those numbers are actually impacting the community is still up for debate.

And perhaps it's the wrong question in the first place. Maybe it should be a case of proving *value* instead of bottom line impact, making a difference to people instead of making a financial entry in a ledger, generating trust instead of revenue. Perhaps the greatest value chaplain managers bring to the job is their faith—their absolute certainty that they are working for a just cause: fair and equal access to care for all, in alignment with their hospital's mission and core values. That faith, paired with their dedication, creativity, and nimbleness, enable them to build trust both inside and outside the walls of the hospital. Because their job description includes a mandate by hospital leadership to be mavericks, free of many of the boundaries facing traditional chaplains and other hospital team members, chaplain managers bring flexibility and in-the-moment adaptability to the job. They are charged with and excel at demonstrating the core values and cultural commitments of their hospital system.

Maybe the reason chaplain managers are trusted by top administration, serve on high-priority hospital teams, are empowered to fully engage with the community, and are considered highly valued staff in times of crisis at the hospital is because they have the courage and commitment to color outside the lines. If it's getting a call in the middle of the night from a jail, they take it. If it's finding shelter for a teenager kicked out of the house, they find it. If it's helping a staff member figure out how to dig out of a financial hole, they do it. If it's understanding great fear, great grief, great hope, and great promise, they hold the space ... and then take the next step. In a word, Jello. In a better word, priceless. Who wouldn't value that kind of person on the team?

> *"Chaplain managers are the people who stand in the gaps of ensuring that the culture of care also has an ear to the needs of the community."*
> — Adam Ridenhour

> *"Being inside and outside the walls of the hospital places us closer to hospital leadership; our opinions are valued and leaders want to hear them."*
> — Dianne Horton

> *"The CHNA was the primary tool to write the grant for transportation services for patients in our county. It's important that we hear the heartbeat of the community, as well as the hospital, and work with our partners in the health department, the pastors, the local ministries, and other organizations to make things happen."*
> — Graylin Carlton

> *"We find that 24/7 crisis spiritual care is the biggest benefit chaplain managers bring to the hospital. Showing up and representing the hospital by supporting patients and families, delivering staff care, and working in the community in times of trouble are highly valued by hospital administration. Chaplain managers are trust revenue: The capital they generate is goodwill and peace of mind."*
> — Emily Viverette

6.

Anglers and Bakers:
Core Competencies and Skills

"In rural communities—everywhere, actually—the general public thinks a preacher can do things other people can't."

— Graylin Carlton

"The chaplain manager role is just like a local pastor. People wander into the hospital off the street and ask for help. And we step up and support."

— Emily Viverette

"We have a lot of autonomy and permission to be creative in what we do. It's not cookie-cutter. Because each campus is different and each community is different, it can't be cookie-cutter."

— Dianne Horton

Mission statements can be inspiring, but they are meaningless without a corporate culture that embraces their values. And while mission statements are often written by the few for the many, the exact opposite is true of culture. In healthy, high-functioning organizations, culture doesn't make people; people make culture.

Like most hospital systems, the Culture Commitments of Atrium Health Wake Forest Baptist Medical Center are powerful because they are the all-important how-tos behind the hospital's mission "To improve health, elevate hope, and advance healing—for all." These Commitments include:

- We create a space where all Belong.
- We work as One Team to make great things happen.
- We earn Trust in all we do.
- We Innovate to better the now and create the future.
- We drive for Excellence—always.[45]

But, what does that actually *look* like?

That's where the chaplain manager comes in. Making these Culture Commitments real for the hospital and community in order to breathe life into its mission is an integral part of the chaplain manager job description—the spark that fires the engine and the fuel that drives their efforts.

Much of the chaplain manager's job is support, paving the way for *others* in the hospital to do *their* jobs: heal. That's what the Culture Commitments are all about—a way of "showing up" in the hospital and the community it serves that promises to do more and be better. It takes a certain kind of person with an exceptional skill set to help the hospital deliver on its commitments—however intangible and hard to make concrete—and more importantly, to get everyone else on the team to do the same. Chaplain managers take these commitments seriously. They specialize in fishes and loaves, turning a little into a feast, bringing action and purpose to noble ideals.

Empowered to Create Change

A Davie County patient was having problems with medication compliance. The patient had been discharged from the hospital with a prescription for a medication that had to be refrigerated, yet had not mentioned to the physician or pharmacist that he did not have a refrigerator. Adam Ridenhour followed up and quickly discovered the problem was not a critical understanding issue. Instead, it was an issue of empowerment: The patient didn't feel comfortable sharing with the provider that he did not have this resource. Ridenhour and the hospital team came alongside and found a way to support the patient: a family member who could safely house the antibiotic in their refrigerator. Chaplain managers are trained to understand that equitably accessible social drivers of health (food, housing, transportation, education, money/jobs, connected language and culture, a healthy environment, and inclusion)[46] are the solid underpinnings of a healthy community. "Because of the partnership with our pharmacy colleagues, we were able to refine our Health Equity Pharmacy Program to ensure there are no barriers to accessing medications once patients leave the emergency department," Ridenhour said.

In the by-the-book hospital world of regulations and standards, the chaplain manager is the unicorn—that rare individual trained (and required)—to move seamlessly between hospital departments, teams, and committees, as well as towns, neighborhoods, agencies, and boards in the communities their hospital serves. By design, the job of chaplain manager is the perfect marriage of objective with subjective, a careful balancing act of more freedom and less liability as they do their work of clinical care, readmissions, and behavioral health. For example, a hospital pharmacist completing a medication requisition is more rigid and tied to a process chart, by design. The function of a chaplain manager is more creative and borderless, yet with the same capacity to improve health outcomes—and even save lives—as the pharmacist. It may just be harder to discern and the improvement seen farther down the road.

Specialist vs. Generalist: A Both-And

But never doubt that the role of a chaplain manager is a catch-22. Their broad skills categorize them as generalists, while their dual role as traditional chaplains makes them more specialists. So, which is it? And, does it even matter?

In his paper, *Beyond Clinical Specificity: A Model of Chaplaincy and Clinical Spiritual Care Within the Shifting Paradigm of Population Health*, Adam Ridenhour suggests considering the unique chaplain manager model through a third lens: specialized generalist or generalized specialist.[9] His argument is persuasive: It takes highly specialized tools and a commitment to establishing community webs of relationships to perform the expansive generalist role of what Ridenhour calls "champions of population health, preventative care, values-based health care, and general community trust."[9]

Perhaps most important of all, by its organic nature the role is highly adaptable and fluid to match the individual chaplain manager's strengths and interests, making partnership absolutely crucial. For example, one chaplain manager may be adept at developing community partnerships while another is better at fundraising; a third excels at initiating new programs while a fourth's background is in counseling. While all chaplain managers have arenas of specialization, the true gift—and challenge—is to use that specialization, girded by the firm foundation of spiritual care, to re-engage a generalist ministry. On the one hand, it's to be a traditional minister and attend board meetings and meet the call to deliver supportive spiritual care, and at the same time, be willing to assume the role of change agent and step into the weeds of workplace violence, ethics, and the mystery that was COVID. Bottom line, while specialists and generalists are very different, the job of the chaplain manager is to blend the two distinct roles into one.

And that's no small task. In a large hospital system, it's normal for teams to be siloed in their efforts: one team doing community work, another team managing behavioral health, others handling congregational work, some working with CPE, and still more involved in spiritual care. Yet the chaplain manager is tasked with it all. The trick—and an integral part of the training of a chaplain manager—is to first take a deep breath and recognize how all those disparate departments are, in truth, working for a common cause, and then shrink that global view to the micro level and assume those various hats on their own hospital campuses.

Of course, context is everything—whether it's the timeless—and yet ever-evolving—needs of a small, rural community or a moment in time whose time has finally come. Ridenhour points out that the chaplain manager model brings to life the founding goal of the original School and Department of Pastoral Care of North Carolina Baptist Hospitals (and the forerunner of the FaithHealth Education Department at Atrium Wake Forest Baptist Hospital), the primary driver of the holistic delivery of health care. For him, that goal is to *be* the healing ministry of Jesus and take seriously the healing of mind, body, and spirit.[9] It doesn't get any more specific—and general—than that.

> "Sometimes the layout of the day depends on the path I take to the mail room. The people I meet along the way are how I figure out where my day is going."
>
> — Dianne Horton

"I think each of the roles that we play has their own value dynamic to bring to the mix: obviously there is the specialized spiritual care and the accompaniment that goes along with it. Where the generalist part comes in is that we are one of a few within the hospital that serves in multiple functions in multiple spaces, with the specificity to listen to patients' and teammates' concerns, but also with a broad enough scope to be on the workplace violence committee at the hospital and the aging committee for our counties. I think there's a big value in not only filling the gaps between social support structures for patients in the community but also helping hold various health system initiatives together too."

— Adam Ridenhour

Professional Standards

However creative and "unboxed" chaplain managers may be, they abide by a set of rigorous common competencies approved by many respected chaplaincy organizations, including Association for Clinical Pastoral Education (ACPE), Association of Professional Chaplains (APC), Canadian Association of Spiritual Care (CASC), National Association of Catholic Chaplains (NACC), and Neshama, Association of Jewish Chaplains (NAJC).

Along with being able to integrate chaplaincy theory with actual spiritual care practice, these competencies include:[47]

- Professional Conduct
    * Identifying their professional strengths and limitations in the delivery of care
    * Articulating how feelings, values, assumptions, culture, and social location affect their professional practice

* Taking care of their own physical, emotional, and spiritual well-being
* Respecting the physical, cultural, emotional, and spiritual boundaries of others
* Appropriately using their professional authority as a chaplain
* Advocating for the people in their care

- Professional Practice Skills
  * Bringing sensitivity, respect, and openness to professional spiritual care relationships
  * Providing effective spiritual support that contributes to the well-being of care recipients, including patients (or same in a non-healthcare setting), their families/friends, and staff
  * Providing care that respects diversity relative to differences in race, culture, gender, sexual orientation, etc.
  * Triaging and managing crises from a spiritual care perspective
  * Providing comfort to those experiencing loss and grief
  * Sharing religious/spiritual resources that are appropriate to care recipients, their spirituality/religion, contexts, and goals
  * Developing, coordinating, and facilitating public/semi-public liturgy appropriate to a range of settings and needs
  * Facilitating care recipient's theological/spiritual/philosophical reflection
  * Facilitating group processes in the provision of spiritual care

* Making and using spiritual assessments to inform chaplain interventions and contribute to interdisciplinary plans of care

* Documenting their own spiritual care accurately, cautiously, and usefully and in the appropriate records

- Organizational Leadership Competencies

    * Promoting the integration of spiritual care into the institution they serve

    * Building and maintaining professional and interdisciplinary relationships

    * Understanding and functioning with their institutional culture and system, including using business best practices appropriate to their role in the organization

    * Advocating for and facilitating ethical decision-making in the workplace

    * Fostering collaborative relationships with community faith leaders and clergy[47]

Chaplain Manager Skills

What does it take to exemplify these conducts, practices, and competencies? Which skills best serve the hospital and its community? How *does* the rubber meet the road in the day-to-day life of a chaplain manager? In her paper, *Building Bridges: Integrating Community Engagement Skills into Clinical Pastoral Education at Atrium Health Wake Forest Baptist,* Emily Viverette states the FaithHealth logic of being savvy, perceptive, and well-informed are vital—understanding the community medical center's culture priorities as well as the local demographics, culture, history, and resources.[12] Having a firm grasp of boundary leadership is important. The ability to embrace leading causes of life (agency, coherence/sense-making, hope, connection, and intergenerativity/blessing) and an abundance mindset versus a scarcity mindset are helpful to communities.[12] Last, seeing with an asset-based lens (the strengths and gifts of a community) instead of the traditional pathology lens is key.[12] Viverette's list of winning attitudes that support FaithHealth logic includes a willingness to work outside the walls of the hospital, being open and trustworthy, feeling a kinship with and invested in the community, and being committed to advocating for the underserved.[12] Viverette's breakdown of chaplain manager skills and competencies falls into clear categories:

- Self-care skills
- Generalist skills
- Partnership skills
    * can identify key partners inside and outside the hospital walls and develop innovative, mutually beneficial partnerships for better health
    * can serve as a translator and/or gatekeeper or boundary leader between the hospital and community it serves in clear, culturally-sensitive ways
- Navigating/Connecting Skills
    * can navigate and discover existing and new community and faith resources (especially food, transportation, behavioral health)
    * able to connect people and organizations with community and congregational resources
    * can find value in and leverage informal relationships for better health

* able to educate the community about FaithHealth
* can represent the hospital at community and faith events, as well as on local boards
* able to understand and relate to medical center leadership

FaithHealth Knowledge Competencies

- Community Medical Center Savvy
  * Understands the medical center mission, culture, and priorities
  * Understands FaithHealth financial logic (the relevance of community benefit and the CHNA, Community Health Needs Assessment)
- Community Savvy
  * Understands the culture, demographics, history, and resources
  * Understands how the community views the medical center
  * Knows the key community stakeholders and their priorities (agencies, congregations, leaders)
  * Grasps the local culture's key disparities and challenges (behavioral health, food, transportation, etc.)

Of course, along with these competencies, skills, and training are the hours of annual continuing education, memberships in professional associations, peer review, exhaustive documentation of good standing, and adherence to a common code of ethics in the field.[11]

It's an impressive list for a role that also demands good instincts, deep faith, an affinity for people, humility, and the courage to be willing to step into the unknown with others every single day.

COVID: UNITY BUILDS COMMUNITY

During the confusion, fear, hardship, and loss of the COVID-19 pandemic, something amazing happened. For the first time, mayors of both little townships in Wilkes County called the community pastors together to be the calming voices during the pandemic. It was an historic event—the first time all the county's Black and white clergy were in a room together to talk about a community problem. After they all arrived, one of the mayors turned to hospital chaplain manager Graylin Carlton and surprised him by asking if he would take the lead and answer questions and advise clergy on how to react. "I thought, wow," Carlton said. "COVID wasn't in the Black community or the white community: It was in our community, everywhere. We had to learn to be innovative, to communicate, to facilitate understanding—which is what chaplain managers do every day. I grew up here, I know these clergy, and I have never seen anything like it in this county. COVID helped us build new relationships, new ties. It brought this community together in a different way, and I was right in the middle of it."

Perhaps that's the chaplain manager's superpower—the ability to be multilingual in a sense, to intuitively know how to be present with a wide variety of constituents. Whether it's discussing the community health needs assessment with a hospital administrator or recruiting a Southern Baptist pastor to mobilize his congregation in a project, relating with a scared patient or speaking truth to power at a tense community meeting, these diverse scenarios all require diverse "languages" and chaplain managers are often the Rosetta Stone of their hospital system. They have the ability to be conversant with people from all walks of life—at work in a team meeting or at prayer in a patient's room during a dark-night-of-the-soul moment. In the effort to straddle these very different worlds, the North Star for chaplain managers is simple: meet people where they are, maintain integrity, honor confidentiality, see others' perspectives while bringing a fresh perspective, and remember that everyone is doing their best in the moment. They are trained to journey with others.

CHAPLAIN MANAGERS:
THE WILL TO CARE, THE POWER TO ACT

Chaplain managers are trusted with people's stories on all levels, without judgment and with complete empathy. That's how they earn trust and respect, that's how they get things done. When an eighteen-year-old teenager walked up to the Davie Medical Center front desk asking for help, Adam Ridenhour didn't hesitate. The boy's intoxicated father had kicked him out of the house for good that morning. The boy had no driver's license, no ID, nothing but the clothes on his back, and no clue about homeless shelters and who to turn to. Because he wasn't a patient, hospital social workers couldn't help. But Ridenhour could. "As chaplain managers, we could step into that gap and help him figure things out," he said. "We worked as a team. I called Graylin about shelters and other possibilities. That's what we do." That same level of care and trust applies to hospital staff. "We have a limited English-speaking person on staff who has worked with the hospital for years and is about to be evicted from their home," Emily Viverette shared. "This person came to us to figure it out and we are the people helping find a way." When a physician, end-of-life patient, and family were at odds about next steps, Graylin Carlton was called in to talk to all parties and facilitate understanding. "We got them to come together to really hear each other, and ultimately, support the patient in the choice of hospice," he said. "It was tough, but it worked out for the best in the end."

Key Takeaways: Go-to Competencies and Skills

While the role of chaplain manager is crucial, it is usually complicated and often nuanced. However, the goal is always the same: Accompany people on whatever journey they are on with compassion and creativity. These ways of being are foundational to success—and job satisfaction.

- **BE organized.** The devil is in the details. Organization is critical to the function—being able to juggle roles, multi-task assignments, and hold multiple spaces at the same time. (Oh yes, and breathe.)
- **BE curious.** Choose to learn continuously—especially about different cultures, ensuring relevance and true service.
- **BE humble.** Make no assumptions regarding need, expectations, and interventions based on the person in front of you.
- **BE discerning.** Self- and situational awareness are key. As the list of people and projects needing support lengthens, it's important to recognize when, where, and how to share gifts and skills. Even a borderless job requires boundaries sometimes—know when to hold 'em and when to fold 'em.
- **BE open and receptive.** Flexibility leads to creative problem-solving, which includes the wisdom to partner with knowledgeable others with complementary skills and talents.
- **BE creative.** Unite the right and left brain to assess the problem and brainstorm innovative solutions.
- **BE nimble.** It's vital to be able to turn on a dime and quickly adapt to rapidly shift sands, evolving inputs, and changing information. Recognize which hat to put on for the job at-hand, how much of the hat to wear, and how long to wear it.

- **BE a good listener.** Hold the space with—and for—others, and maintain confidentiality. Deep listening applies to functional goals as well. Listen for the role required in a given situation: whether it's working on a CHNA with hospital colleagues, advocating for a patient's wishes about advanced directives with family, or serving on a community team for the collective good.
- **BE aware.** Context is always going to shape the role and the goal, informing where and how to move forward. Meeting people where they are is paramount.

"We are the bridge, connecting the dots, and it comes at us from all angles. It's a constant give and take."
— Dianne Horton

"Chaplain managers are really good at remaining grounded in their values and being guided by those values no matter what comes up. Because they are trained not to be swayed by the forces around them, they are able to maintain a keen sense of the next right thing."
— Emily Viverette

Sometimes we are in places we need to be ... but don't want to be. Still, we show up. It's all about commitment.
— Graylin Carlton

The role of chaplain manager is empowering, meaningful, satisfying, and even enjoyable. But never doubt that it is a holy calling. They are also absolutely dedicated. Yes, it's hard. Yes, the hours can be long. Yes, it's a constant to have to come up with another fish or a fresh loaf. Again. And yes, the need is endless, broad, deep, and oftentimes daunting. A chaplain manager often feels like the little girl pitching the starfish strewn along the beach back into the water. Admonished by her father for taking on such a huge, hopeless task that couldn't possibly make a dent, she quietly yet firmly responded, "I made a difference to *that* one." Like that little girl, chaplain managers agree: to make a difference to even one person is important ... life-changing ... soul-satisfying. It's a commitment worth making.

7.

The Cup that Runneth Over:
Challenges, Lessons, The Future

"There's an identity crisis all around: in the church, in western health care, in population health, in chaplaincy. We're all searching. Something has changed and we can all point philosophically to what this is in each of our circles. I think we are at that point in the change cycle where something can really take shape and we can do something new and innovative."

— Adam Ridenhour

"For me, it's all about access. And we did it: Now my hospital has a cardiac rehab and a heart center, we've expanded our ED services, and we want an oncology/hematology center here. That's why I'm still doing this. Three out of five days, I want to say 'I'm done' but I feel it's important that I'm here. I want to help the community—whether it's to build a Rosenwald school or get a patient to their appointment. This is the real world and this is a real-life experience. I can either step away or make sure lack of access doesn't happen to another person ever again."

— Graylin Carlton

The beauty of the FaithHealth model is that it is a catch-all space for walking alongside people who have fallen through the cracks of the social support structure in a relationship of trust and support. Chaplain managers are those professionals who stand in the vacuum with their arms wide open, ready to catch those who fall, armed with clear parameters for what can be done, what can't, and how to distinguish the difference ... quickly. The reasons a person chooses the calling of chaplain manager are as varied as the individual: a testament to faith, an expression of love, an act for social justice, the desire to heal.

But that doesn't mean there aren't challenges, lessons learned, and recommendations for ways to do things smarter, better, faster. Despite the many issues, their passion shows up in their values and keeps them moving forward. The wind beneath the wings of the chaplain manager's unshakeable commitment to true equity and inclusion are the usual: zeal, dedication, and compassion (with a lot of stubbornness, sticktoittiveness, and yes, bravery).

Challenges

> *"Challenges and opportunities are the same thing. It's about resources, trust, nonjudgment, and education."*
> — Adam Ridenhour

Like all clergy, chaplain managers are on the front lines when times turn tough. Unlike clergy, chaplain managers are based in hospitals—often the end of the line for catastrophes and where the rubber meets the road when it comes to hope and help. But not all disasters are hurricanes, mass shootings, car wrecks, and industrial accidents. Because chaplain managers are also solidly based in the community they live in, they confront the sociological challenges that deeply impact local people, especially the underserved.

Historically, these include poverty; racism; hate; big pharma's role in creating and fueling the opioid crisis (an enormous issue facing rural communities);[48] and eugenics efforts, a form of racism that inaccurately espouses that the human race can be improved through selective breeding. A false belief still active today in the US and around the world, at its core eugenics is about discrimination, ableism, and colonialism. It includes practices such as involuntary sterilization, forced institutionalization, ostracization, and the destruction of marginalized ethnic minorities, those with disabilities, and the LGBTQ+ community.[49]

The most recent health challenge brought the US—the entire planet—to its knees. The COVID-19 pandemic and the ensuing politicizing of the deadly disease killed millions around the world, and more than a million (and counting) in the US,[50] disproportionately affecting people of color, those with comorbidities, the elderly, and the underserved.[50,51,52]

The Opioid Crisis

The end of the twentieth century brought with it one of the most devastating public health crises in the US: the opioid catastrophe. According to the CDC, from 1999 till 2021, 645,000 people in the US died of an opioid overdose (both prescription and illicit drugs); six times more people died in 2021 than 1999. There was a more than 16 percent increase in the number of drug overdose deaths from 2020 to 2021, with 220 people dying every day in 2021—75 percent of them due to opioids. This was a chilling 15 percent increase over the previous year.[53]

Misuse of opioids has adversely affected the labor market, contributing to absenteeism, workplace accidents, and loss of staff due to incarceration, disability, or death.[54] Each year dependence, misuse, and overdose of opioids costs the US $35 billion for health care, $14.8 billion for criminal justice measures, and $92 billion in lost workplace productivity.[55] According to the CDC, the 2017 economic cost of the US opioid crisis was $1.021 trillion ($471 billion for opioid use disorder and $550 billion for fatal opioid overdose).[56] In 2020, costs had skyrocketed to $1.5 trillion, up 37 percent from 2017.[57]

Despite the public outcry and media coverage, opioid overdoses remain a serious public health problem. Many attribute that to COVID-19 and the whiplash-fast jerk of the public and scientific attention away from the opioid epidemic to the coronavirus pandemic. Yet it's estimated 1.2 million *more* people in the US and Canada will die from opioid overdose by 2030,[50,58] many of them in reaction to the isolation and fear caused by the new crisis, COVID, as well as the same-old story: a continuing lack of access to prevention and quality care. While addiction care is often separate from mainstream medical care, it is also hit-and-miss in terms of quality and plagued by social stigma and barriers to care.

Enter the chaplain manager. They are trained to go to those places of discomfort where others prefer not to travel and deliver support that is insightful as well as compassionate: whether it's as simple as using the term "substance use disorder" instead of the judgmental "substance abuse" or the more complicated move to step into the gap in the moment to help a congregation and a family understand the complexities of a disease that impacts not just the person but entire communities—especially in the rural south.

MEETING PEOPLE WHERE THEY ARE

There is a raging wildfire spreading across Small Town America, and nothing has stopped it yet. It's substance abuse. According to a Rand study released in 2024, nearly half of all Americans know someone who has died of a drug overdose; and a third of those say their lives have been forever changed by an OD death.[59] In 2022, more than 109,000 people died from an overdose; 1.1 million since the year 2000.[59] That's a lot of loss. It's one that Graylin Carlton sees every week in rural Wilkes County. Despite the magnitude of this public health challenge, substance-users in rural areas still face deep stigma, with few people to talk to about addiction and the problems it causes. Carlton is one of those few because he is trained to see substance abuse as a disease and not a choice to be frowned upon. While many local pastors feel prayer and conversion are the best ways to resolve an addiction problem, chaplain managers intervene in communities, homes, and churches with conversation and education, helping all parties better understand the issue. Because of limited mental health services in smaller and rural communities, professional chaplain managers, with their background in and understanding of mental health, can be a great resource. "We're trained to address the issue differently from a pastor's perspective," Carlton said. "It's still spiritual, just not from that point of view. We're taught to meet the person right where they are. It's not about recruiting for the church; it's about meeting spiritual needs."

THE COVID PANDEMIC

"When a pastor tells a congregant, what does that doctor know?, the entire community suffers. There's a health concern in the community and how can they trust the health system? This was especially prevalent in smaller rural communities during COVID."
— Graylin Carlton

"We sit in the space of the unknown. We work to ensure the patient is not alone, they are not separate from the health team."
— Adam Ridenhour

It was a frightening time—especially for smaller rural hospitals. In the middle of the opioid crisis came COVID-19. The virus was deadly; the data and recommendations, like the virus, were rapidly changing; North Carolina, like other states, was mandating shelter-in-place and social-distancing measures; the hospital was encouraging people to get the vaccine; and then the worst happened: The pandemic became a political football, once again dividing the country. But it was not a game people were losing—it was their lives.

What started as a snowball became an unstoppable avalanche of social, health, and economic destruction for many, making the job of chaplain manager even more difficult, because they were on the front line representing the health care system. While dealing with the misinformation and mistrust was frustrating, it was also easy to see why people were scared and upset. It was the same-old story: The virus, like opioids, was disproportionately affecting people of color, the marginalized, the old, and the sick.[60,61] Yes, they were chaplains, but they were chaplains who worked for the hospital. Once again, the bridge between the two worlds of health care system and community was widening. Once again, trust was vital—something chaplain managers were expert at building ... *and* proving.

CARING THROUGH COVID

The COVID-19 pandemic was a rural hospital's worst nightmare. Despite emergency preparations and planning, the trauma of a system bursting at the seams with the sick and dying was compounded by ignorance, supply chain challenges, lack of resources, staffing problems, mistrust, job losses, fear, stress, anger, and grief. COVID was a quicksand of not knowing what you didn't know—and people were sinking fast. The politicizing of the pandemic elevated protective masking to a human rights violation—while at the same time denying the human right to life to people who caught the disease from those who refused to take basic recommended safety precautions. It was a time of creating special waivers for those refusing to mask, requests for religious exemptions for masking, medical providers being accused of murder after a COVID death, and broken hearts when families couldn't be in the rooms of the sick and dying, as well as the new infants and patients in treatment. Because smaller campuses were more intimate and staff knew each other better, tension was especially high around the vaccination requirements. Chaplain managers stood between staff who wanted to be vaccinated and those who didn't—*each* assuming the chaplain was on *their* side. That's actually the beauty of the chaplain manager role: the ability to walk the line in between, treating everyone the same, regardless of their beliefs, staying in the middle as everyone went through the hard times of COVID together. "Helping people feel heard, appreciated, and respected is important," said Emily Viverette. "But it's equally important to name the discrepancy and speak one's own truth. That's also part of the chaplain manager role." It's a fine line to walk, and Adam Ridenhour feels chaplain managers live *hard* in that line with their constituents: teammates, patients, the community, and local elected leaders. Especially during COVID. "How do you stay in the place of caring when people won't let you care, if they kick you out of the room?" Ridenhour said. "Chaplain managers are in the business of showing up—showing up for patients, family, the medical team, pastors, hospital staff—all of whom live in the community and go to the churches, and suddenly everyone's talking about not wanting to wear masks. In times of trouble, this is where the point of trust comes in. Chaplain managers are expert at holding the space. Being a trusted person in the community spheres of patients, staff, and other agencies allows us to step into places of accompaniment rather than opposition, walking alongside folks—not in front of or behind them. Because we had cultivated these trusting relationships over time, when we were in the thick of things we could help inform decisions regarding community outreach."

COVID was devastating for the health care system and workers. But it was also an opportunity for institutional innovation and adaptation. During COVID, traditional spiritual care moved front-and-center again. Chaplain managers shifted to virtual and telephone pastoral care with patients and families because of limited hospital visitation and rapidly diminishing supplies of necessary PPE, such as masks and hand sanitizer.[9] They devised creative ways for families unable to enter rooms to "be with" sick loved ones—either via virtual gatherings on devices or through a window while on the phone. They orchestrated video-conferenced baptisms and good-byes. They instituted regular prayer, meditation, counseling, and personal check-ins with maxed—and stressed—out staff who were heroically doing their jobs while battling panic, anxiety, depression, exhaustion, grief, and gut-wrenching fear.[9] Referrals to the hospital Employee Emergency Fund (EEF), which chaplain managers oversee, skyrocketed.[9]

While "the world stopped," community engagement did not. It became absolutely vital. Because of the intentional development of networks of trust over time, chaplain managers played a critical role in educating clergy about the evolving medical and scientific evidence, best practices, and recommendations for health and safety to share with their congregations. They also worked with churches to offer safe shelters for hospital staff needing a bed for the night, too afraid to go home to their families.[9] There was even a time when a group home for persons with disabilities was feeling isolated and missing the church experience. They invited a chaplain manager to bring "church" to them via video conference. Chaplain managers stood in the midst of the chaos and fear, lack and hopelessness, and found ways to reconnect people separated by trauma and drama to each other—*and* themselves.

Lessons Learned

> *"An important part of The How of the chaplain manager role is listening and watching for what's missing: whether it's people at a table or a topic no one wants to address or denial of problems; for instance, hearing someone say, again, that there is not a homelessness problem in the community. Being able to name it, lift it up and call attention to things, those are chaplain skills: naming the elephants in the room in communities and spaces when it's not popular."*
> — Adam Ridenhour

> *"It's because of the randomness and chaos that can sometimes occur in health care settings that chaplain managers must be allowed to function in creative ways."*
> — Emily Viverette

> *"It's being able to adjust on the fly—code-switching, or some people just are not going to want you there. I've learned whatever it takes to help others, as long as it's aboveboard and we're doing it the right way, I'll do it."*
> — Graylin Carlton

> *"You have to be politically savvy."*
> — Dianne Horton

True growth comes from challenges and change. Lessons learned often become the rules of the road ... unless you're a chaplain manager. Because that role includes speaking truth, there is a constant tension between doing the job and doing what's right. While the foundational competencies of deep listening, empathy, advocacy, a heart for service, and a passion for social justice are important, the tried-and-true, road-tested skills of political savvy, balance, flexibility, and adaptability are absolutely crucial. Those skills often ignite from baptism by fire—being in the moment with a person in trouble, navigating a tough situation, or working to mend a broken system. No matter what is happening, perhaps the most important lesson of all is one most people learn in kindergarten—to watch out for each other, take care of each other, help each other. That way of approaching the work undergirds everything chaplain managers do—it is who they are at their core. But these other lessons can help too.

About Change

> **Adam Ridenhour:** Since things will change, you need to be ready for it and able to accept it. Whether it's a positive change, a negative change, or something that has nothing to do with us but still impacts the overall environment around us, being able to stretch and flex yet continue to know what our purpose is and what the needs are and adapt those to whatever environment we're in, is part of the dance that we do.
>
> **Graylin Carlton:** Before, I had a much narrower vision. Now my vision is wider. Our training through CPE (Clinical Pastoral Education) opened up lanes—entire avenues—for me on how to deal, be present, listen, and reflect ... *then* act.
>
> **Dianne Horton:** Sometimes the only answer we have is, I don't know. I remember getting a call to help out a patient needing a ramp. I tried all my usual sources, an aging ministry, senior services, and then a congregation I could always count on for help. The gentleman who ran the church program was no longer able to take on that kind of work and no one else had stepped up in his place. It was so hard telling the patient's navigator that I didn't have a way to fix this problem. And when the navigator asked me, well, who are you going to call next?, having to say, I don't know, was hard. It hurt me that we couldn't do it.

About Relationships

Emily Viverette: The real nuance of this work is that chaplain managers have to be so discerning as to which faith organizations are willing to meet people where they are. Of course, some faith organizations are only interested in helping people who think, act, and look like them, and that's OK—that's the politics of faith in some churches and institutions. But it's an important part of our work to find those *other* faith organizations who are willing to support those outside of their congregations and ideology. It can be disappointing when a church seems all-in but really only wants to help people who believe the way they do—their own members.

Adam Ridenhour: I'm in a rebuilding phase with my faith partnerships, starting over with many of the denominations that I traditionally have partnered with. Many leaders have left and these churches are now being served by new pastors that I don't know and who are new to the area. We're moving along, we are past the hump of COVID in terms of our reengagement with each other. But for that denomination, it is rediscovering in the midst of their own identity crisis how we can be together in this community missionally.

Graylin Carlton: While I would not visit a church for counseling, I *would* come to the hospital and talk to the chaplain, because what chaplains do is look at situations through a different lens. The church is failing in America and chaplain managers are doing things that really help. If you need help, people say, go to the church. But churches have a different criteria and rules for getting you gas, food, transportation assistance, etc. We don't do that. We help, regardless. We meet people right where they are, as they are. And that's why it's going to work. We're moving to a point where we are going to need more of what we're doing as the world changes and becomes more colorful, less white, and a more blended society.

Dianne Horton: There was a conversation I'll never forget, when the person was so out of touch and judgmental. I don't want those partners. And when that person said, don't call me, you know, I thought, I won't. So I work to find partners who are nonjudgmental, have a heart for people, understand what it means to have a need, and truly want to help.

Graylin Carlton: When I came here, there were people who would not come to this hospital for all the reasons of mistrust and fear and suspicion. And I feel like I've been a conduit in the community. I'm doing my work and now everyone in our community feels like they can come to the hospital and be served. It wasn't like that before. Of course, they didn't have chaplaincy before either. The lack of a chaplain in the community was detrimental; having a chaplain has helped build those bridges and restore trust.

About Personal Skills and Capacities

Emily Viverette: It's important to recognize your own competence and limits of your competence. A big piece of the training is knowing when we've met our limits: We can't help because we actually don't know what we're doing. And if you don't know what you're doing, it may be more harmful.

Adam Ridenhour: All of us have various motivations—some things really motivate us and speak to our souls and feed our passions. And some hats we wear we have less motivation for, but we have to remember it all feeds a bigger purpose.

Graylin Carlton: After completing my training, I thought, I'm going to be able to go to a room and pray with people and help them through their bereavement. But then, a part of this is taking chaplaincy outside the walls and thinking out of the box. We get to define that. I never thought I would be involved in all these boards and do all these assignments and start a transportation program. FaithHealth gave us the leeway to come to our communities and identify what needed to take place, and then it stood behind us, encouraged us, and gave us the help we needed to make it happen.

Dianne Horton: It's important to have a community, because it can feel isolating in a small hospital by yourself. It can be easy to beat yourself up figuring out job demands and priorities. It can be busy with so many hats to wear and so much to do. I've learned that a community of peers can relieve those worries and inspire me.

Adam Ridenhour: How do you make spiritual care rounds but also do twenty-seven other things at the same time? The ability to triage needs is important in this job, because initially it can be very overwhelming. Also, quantitatively, it can be hard to measure our success, to broaden the lens beyond spiritual care and specializations to include the business and administrative parts of the work. You have to be very creative to figure out your own systems.

CARING THROUGH THE GROWING PAINS

While Dianne Horton has found a quiet purpose, the ability to listen to and keep the stories for others and a passion for social justice in her job as a chaplain manager, the day-to-day challenges can be big. Her on-the-grow hospital is committed to being well-connected, present, supportive, and engaged with the community, with hospital leaders on many different boards and at key local events. But with a merger and larger footprint came growing pains. Before the merger, the hospital could simply write a check to support long-time favorite community fundraisers. Now, formal sponsorship is required. Nonprofits requesting funds must complete a registration process through a hospital website, write a grant proposal, and justify a budget and spending. Flaws in the online system regularly thwart access, prompting a flood of phone calls to hospital personnel ill-equipped to help agencies hitting a wall navigating the new process. "The bigness of the system can unnecessarily complicate things and depersonalize the role of the hospital in the community," she said. "What I learn from the people I work with day-to-day informs my decisions and provides me the knowledge I need to speak truth to power." Complicated processes are particularly problematic in rural communities, according to Graylin Carlton. "No matter how big the system gets, we're still in Small America, we're still rural hospitals" he said. "Having someone on the hospital side say, 'Hey, you didn't cross my t,' makes it harder to get people the help, the transportation, the access they need when they need it. That makes our jobs more difficult. Rural hospitals deserve our services, but as mergers happen, systems change, and hospital units are closed, it gets harder. When centers close and services move to other locations, neighbors can no longer drop by the hospital to visit, to pick up someone who's been discharged, to see the new baby. It changes the community. It damages access, it damages relationships, and bottom line, it damages health. Part of our job is to maintain that sense of community."

BOUNDARIES, NOT BORDERS

Chaplain managers are similar to local pastors in that they are paid to do the job of ministry. But the chaplain manager's autonomy and empowerment often lead to an expansion of that calling. New projects, new boards to serve on, and new ways to help others increase the workload and expand the job, sometimes exponentially. Adam Ridenhour's interests led him to dive in to patient care. An area of special concern to him as a credentialed counselor was the support of patients with mental and behavioral health needs. In a perfect world, Ridenhour would love to see holistic support, where the health system partners with faith communities, educational institutions, law enforcement, parks and recreation departments, and others to play a role in the mental health care of community members. He dreams of a day when health care can shift from working upstream from acute crises to delivering preventive support structures that promote overall health, emotional self-regulation and resilience. "Right now, it just won't work, he said. "When you're juggling community engagement, the day-to-day emergencies, and staff care, there's just not enough capacity. Learning how to draw boundaries of white lines, yellow lines, and dotted lines of your capacity in the moment is still something we're learning. I'm still working on it." Graylin Carlton has learned to relax with the many hats he wears. "We do whatever the day brings," he said. "Some days, it's hard because I'm needed all day long in the emergency department or the ICU. Other days I'm out in the community. Yes, there are certain things I need to do, but then I bump against something more important or most needed at the time—and I do that instead. I've learned to be more flexible."

"Walking that line of making sure we have some congruency **and** *uniqueness at the same time is important."*

— Adam Ridenhour

"I think I've probably been to places that other people say, I wouldn't go there. But I think that's a part of the ugly ministry we have to do. I think Jesus's ministry was ugly. He goes to eat at Zacchaeus's house. Nobody likes the guy and they say, 'You're gonna eat at the house of the rich tax collector and sinner? Why don't you come here instead? I'm your friend.' But Jesus went—and he made a big difference. Zacchaeus changed. So yeah, I've been those places. Sometimes it's said, 'That colored chaplain really helped me.' It doesn't anger me. I'm a Black man in a county that's 97 percent white. Am I disappointed that people still see things that way? Yes, but it doesn't anger me, because I understand it."

— Graylin Carlton

In a Perfect World ...

> *"The sky's the limit? Funds would be easier to access, because a lot of the problems people have, I know money's not the answer to everything, but it's the answer to a lot of things."*
> — Dianne Horton

> *"This job is like being a pastor of a small church. Sometimes it's a wing and a prayer—you fake it till you make it. You're always behind the eight ball and having to rely on your inner gifts and Spirit to guide you. However, the smaller the facility, the larger the impact a chaplain can make in terms of community and health outcomes."*
> — Emily Viverette

> *"You have to be very relational. You can't be timid and you can't let 'no' hold you back. And you've got to be, I wouldn't say multicultural, but you got to be able to just fit in where you get in."*
> — Graylin Carlton

In terms of the work of chaplain managers, the problem and the solution are often the same thing. Chaplain managers do what they do because there is a vacuum waiting to be filled with all the things they care about and they have permission to operate in that vacuum with flexibility and creativity. On the other hand, it's a really big vacuum and that permission to be flexible and get creative can be all-consuming—*and* time-consuming. The old adage is true: If you want a job done well, ask a busy person to do it. Chaplain managers are busy people. While they are extensively trained and come to the job as expert professionals gifted with the skills and talents of being nimble, adjusting quickly, switching codes adeptly, and staying centered in their purpose and their truth, sometimes, it's just not enough. More is needed.

The Wish List

Dianne Horton: I wish there was less red tape because there are people who have the heart to help, but within this big system, things get complicated. For instance, with transportation, there's insurance and liability and other legal considerations to figure out. I'd like it to be easier so more people can participate.

Adam Ridenhour: Some things can be a long uphill battle. Early asset-mapping in my county indicated a need for a lot of community infrastructure because we didn't have those resources. I'm still fighting for transportation: There is still not a local government-assisted transportation program in the county and we've been ringing that bell since 2013.

Graylin Carlton: In many of our African-American Baptist churches, if you want things done, the women do it. But I can't approach the women. I have to approach the pastors and they decide if they want the women to do it. That can make it difficult for me to help my community.

Dianne Horton: A question that is often raised in my work is how do we bring about systemic change? For example, what must be done to eliminate the need for our own EEF (employee emergency fund)? I'd like to be a part of a movement to analyze earnings, assess who is constantly tapping the fund, and then right-size salaries. It's time for conversations with the right people to address this kind of social justice change.

Adam Ridenhour: The job title can be a struggle in describing our role, especially in the community. A different title that more adequately expresses what we're doing could help. I do a lot of work with our pharmacy equity program, and explaining why a chaplain is calling to talk about a patient's access to medicines is one extra layer that can be hard for my colleagues to work through. I'm not sure if it builds trust or throws up a red flag. But in other places, the chaplain name is an asset because, in this part of the world, it is connected to that trust in faith leaders.

The Future of Chaplain Managers

"We have to know how to be present with the hospital administrator in discussing community health needs assessments. We need to know how to talk to the Southern Baptist pastor. We need to know how to talk to the scared patient. These are all different languages and we have to be well-versed in all of them, because that's how we earn the trust and the respect."
— Dianne Horton

"The future of chaplaincy is more than prayers at the bedside."
— Graylin Carlton

Serving an integral role on the hospital administrative team, having key administrative roles in community organizations, and being a part of important strategic initiatives in the community all have one thing in common: the ability to think outside the traditional chaplaincy box and imagine what could be, with all its power and purpose and promise of doing real good in the world.

THE VIEW FROM THE CRYSTAL BALL

Adam Ridenhour: How do you bolster spiritual care and the relationships, trust, and support that our role offers our patients, staff members, and community? Some of us are working on developing a system for a new model looking at what we can accomplish collectively vs. the one-offs. What excites me is the beauty and challenges of being able to tailor projects and resources to the specific needs of a community and having an organized structure that makes sense in *all* communities. I also wonder if chaplaincy will evolve to where it encompasses less specific spiritual care and more of that re-befriending of congregations and not-for-profits that once accomplished the community work. I think with the transition of community engagement to encompass larger areas, there's going to be a gap between what was community engagement, what is population health, and where we fit in the middle: There's an opportunity for us to grow into that space.

Emily Viverette: If I were to paint an ideal, it would be that the role of chaplain manager is valued enough to add local support in the form of a community health worker working alongside them. Chaplain managers wear a lot of hats and have many responsibilities—it's a real juggling act and can be arduous. I also think the future will bring new ways of looking at silos. Medicine in general is learning that we have to stay out of silos. Even spiritual care has developed its own silos over the past thirty years or so. Now we're learning more about the importance of integration and I'm hopeful that will continue.

Dianne Horton: The role of innovation is going to be important in the future, especially in the next five years or so as we continue to step into those places of the most need and think outside the box. I worry that if we start to structure ourselves in ways that look like a Jack-in-the-box or cookie-cutter, we'll lose the beauty of what we can offer. Communication is crucial. Our reporting structure has a dotted line to the president of our hospitals and we should use that. Being in communication with our leader, having regular meetings, checking in, making sure they are our aware of our activities is a good way to continue to get innovative things done.

Graylin Carlton: The future of chaplaincy is more than prayers at the bedside. In one day I had three referrals for outside help: one patient who's being discharged needs a stand-up walker and can't afford it, a patient who needs to get to the cancer center and doesn't have gas money for the car, and a patient discharged back into the community and it's cold out and there's no propane to heat the house. These are real stories that we deal with on a day-to-day basis. And so I think in the future our role is going to be more of that than saying a prayer and going back to the office and shutting the door.

Adam Ridenhour: I think that with traditional chaplains in spiritual care, the care that chaplains provide has been focused inside the hospital with in-patients. I think the crystal ball for the future of chaplaincy is a change to a model of receiving more referrals for patients in need. I'm working with a patient who was coming in for physical therapy and the therapist found out that the person can't work because of the medical crisis requiring therapy, which means no income and no food in the house. That's where we can come in. Another example is a patient coming in for medicines for mental health and trying to set up an appointment for a psych visit, but he has no phone number and no access points. So, we're trying to get creative with problem-solving by noting on his chart a pre-referral to chaplaincy and the pharmacy equity program, which gets him the meds he needs. So, it's not another wait and see, we're not starting over every time. I like helping people who fall through the cracks and the geeky constructive part of figuring out how to make the system work for them.

"A lot has changed with this living human web of divinity schools, public health departments, health care systems, and nonprofit organizations. And while the idea of Christian institutionalization of forming hospitals, creating retirement homes, and building children's homes is out the window, it's time for a recalling of that institutional element. I think there should be an active and not just hypothetical call to reengage symbiotic denominations and other partners to effect change and team up to provide services to real people with real problems."

— Adam Ridenhour

"For me, social justice, treating all fairly, is informed by my faith, which I bring to my role as chaplain manager. It's about value. That is its value. It's valuing human life. It's valuing community health, it's valuing the dignity and sacredness of human life."
— Dianne Horton

"That's where the ministry part, the selfless part comes in. Lots of the things I do is because they are beneficial to the patient and the community and it's the right thing to do. That's why I do what I do: this right thing and the next right thing and the next right thing, and then you look around and think, OMG, I have a lot to do."
— Graylin Carlton

Uniting Faith and Health in the Service of All

The work of chaplain managers proves their value proposition over and over: Spiritual care is a worthy—and priceless—ally in today's value-based health care arena. Their work to activate the FaithHealth model centers on making sure people go through the right health care door at the right time, ready to be treated and never alone. They believe in right-sizing the healing pyramid that recognizes most health and well-being happen in the community and not the hospital. They work for equal and fair access to health care for everyone—*every* one. Chaplain managers ensure patients not only get regular health care appointments but also are able to *get to* those appointments instead of having to seek emergency treatment at the hospital ED. They prevent everyday people from falling between the cracks—and lend a helping hand if they stumble. They live into a way of being that focuses on community strengths and gifts, keeps an abundance mindset, and aligns with the Leading Causes of Life. All of these are cornerstones of the FaithHealth model—and they all make sense.

From a financial perspective, the FaithHealth model and chaplain manager role save the hospital and the local economy money. It puts resources where they belong—in maintaining health and well-being and preventing disease, which aligns with the goals of the ACA, Medicare, and Medicaid. The nation's health care system is very complex and difficult to navigate. Having trusted professionals embedded within the system that citizens can reach out to furthers the health, economic, justice, humanitarian, and spiritual goals of communities. Being that trusted resource, the bridge, is "The Why" for many people entering the field.

Faith-full and committed to being the hands and feet of love and compassion in the world, chaplain managers willingly, gladly, and capably walk side-by-side with patients along their life journeys ... because true and long-lasting health is about life, *not* hospitals. Yesterday or today, the job is a both-and: building a culture of trust and excellence to safely and equitably bring people into the care of the hospital and using that same trust and excellence to bring good health practices and access into the community.

> *"I love my job. It's my mission to step into the gaps and messiness that our most vulnerable patients find themselves in and tailor support and care to meet those specific needs as they arise. It may be serving a spiritual need with counseling or a physical need like providing transportation. I'm lucky to have the freedom to think outside the box, to step into whatever role best helps people, and address areas of need both inside and outside the walls of the hospital."*
>
> — Adam Ridenhour

"I think the education and training that we have as chaplains—especially the competencies that we meet to be board-certified—equip us to do this job and do it well. We're here to help people in need get away from the judgment, and the 'If you want this meal, then you have to come hear a sermon and a song.' Ministry is broad. As chaplains we've settled ourselves in a category of that broader concept of ministry. But still, we're doing it because there's a call."

— Dianne Horton

"This job is like emotions, up and down every day. We've been through COVID, we have times when it's really lonely, we get beat up a lot, and you get to wondering if all this stuff of going out talking to people and being on boards is really important. Does anybody care or notice? At the recent Christmas tree lighting event, a local organization told me they had some extra money and wanted to donate it to FaithHealth, because they believed in the cause. Well, it was $55,000. That makes you feel good. I didn't ask for this, it just came. I'm so grateful that people in Wilkes County realize we're here to help **all** people. That's why I do this."

— Graylin Carlton

References

I. Introduction

1. Jain, Sachin H. Missed Appointments, Missed Opportunities: Tackling The Patient No-Show Problem. Forbes.com. Oct. 6, 2019. Accessed January 10, 2024. https://www.forbes.com/sites/sachinjain/2019/10/06/missed-appointments-missed-opportunities-tackling-the-patient-no-show-problem/?sh=447d96ce573b

2. Wolfe, Mary K., McDonald, Noreen C., and Holmes, G. Mark. American Journal of Public Health. Transportation Barriers to Health Care in the United States: Findings From the National Health Interview Survey, 1997. May 6, 2020. Accessed January 10, 2024. https://pubmed.ncbi.nlm.nih.gov/32298170/

3. Gunderson, Gary. The Missing Space. FaithHealth Magazine. Spring, 2013. https://faithhealth.org/wp-content/uploads/2014/01/FaithHealth-Magazine-Spring-2013-Web.pdf

4. Long, Katelyn N.G., Symons, Xavier, Vanderweele, Tyler, J., Balboni, Tracy A., Rosmarin, David H., Puchalski, Christina, Cutts, Teresa, Gunderson, Gary R., et al. Spirituality As A Determinant Of Health: Emerging Policies, Practices, And Systems. Health Affairs. June 2024. Accessed August 1, 2024. https://www.healthaffairs.org/doi/full/10.1377/hlthaff.2023.01643

5. Simmons, Tracy. Interest in chaplaincy grows as the role expands to serve more in society. Faith & Leadership. April 30, 2024. Accessed July 10, 2024. https://faithandleadership.com/interest-chaplaincy-grows-the-role-expands-serve-more-society

6 Hospital Closures Threaten Patient Access to Care as Hospitals Face a Range of Rising Pressures. American Hospital Association. September 8, 2022. https://www.aha.org/press-releases/2022-09-08-new-aha-report-finds-rural-hospital-closures-threaten-patient-access-care

7. Condon, Alan. States with the most rural hospital closures. Becker's Healthcare: Hospital CFO Report. November 28, 2023. Accessed July 12, 2024.

https://www.beckershospitalreview.com/finance/states-with-the-most-rural-hospital-closures.html

8. James, Julia. Nonprofit Hospitals' Community Benefit Requirements. Health Affairs. February 25, 2016. Accessed July 10, 2024. https://www.healthaffairs.org/content/briefs/nonprofit-hospitals-community-benefit-requirements#:~:text=Under%20the%20%22community%20benefit%22%20standard%2C%20spending%20that%20promotes,determining%20what%20activities%20and%20services%20constituted%20community%20benefit.

2. The FaithHealth Chaplaincy Model: A Framework for Caring

9. Ridenhour, Adam. Beyond Clinical Specificity: A Model of Chaplaincy and Clinical Spiritual Care Within the Shifting Paradigm of Population Health. 2022. Dissertation, Duke University Divinity School. Accessed March 6, 2024. https://dukespace.lib.duke.edu/items/040bae67-d878-455a-8ccf-f739fdee8f00

10. Magnan, Sanne. Social Determinants of Health 101 for Health Care: Five Plus Five. National Academy of Medicine. October 9, 2017. Accessed July 9, 2024. https://nam.edu/social-determinants-of-health-101-for-health-care-five-plus-five/

11. Hood, C.M., Gennuso, K.P., Swain, G.R., and Catlin, B.B. County health rankings: Relationships between determinant factors and health outcomes. American Journal of Preventive Medicine. 50(2):129 135. 2016. Accessed July 18, 2024. https://doi.org/10.1016/j.amepre.2015.08.024

12. Viverette, Emily Bennett. Building Bridges: Integrating Community Engagement Skills into Clinical Pastoral Education at Atrium Health Wake Forest Baptist. (Hood Theological Seminary, DMin Project) Salisbury, NC, 2022. Accessed March 6, 2024.

13. Leading Causes of Life website. Accessed March 6, 2024. http://www.leading-causes.com/uploads/2/0/2/3/20235431/leading_causes_of_life_-_revisited1.pdf

14. Gunderson, Gary and Pray, Larry. Leading Causes of Life: Five Fundamentals to Change the Way You Live Your Life. Abingdon Press. January 1, 2008. Accessed March 6, 2024.

15. Kenington, Tammy. What Is Hope and Why Do We Need It So Badly. Christianity.com. June 17, 2021. Accessed July 10, 2024. https://www.christianity.com/wiki/christian-terms/what-is-hope-and-why-do-we-need-it-so-badly.html

16. Bentorah, Chaim. Word Study—Hope or Certainty. April 1, 2014. Accessed July 10, 2024. https://www.chaimbentorah.com/2014/04/word-study-hope-certainty/

17. What is the Christian's hope? Got Questions Ministry. Accessed July 10, 2024. https://www.gotquestions.org/hope-Bible.html

18. Cochrane, James and Gunderson, Gary. Barefoot Guide to Mobilizing Religious Health Assets for Transformation, Volume 3. Accessed March 6, 2024

19. DePaul University Asset-based Community Development Institute (abcd Institute). 2024. Accessed March 8, 2024. https://resources.depaul.edu/abcd-institute/Pages/default.aspx

20. UCLA Center for Health Policy Research: Section 1. Asset Mapping. Accessed March 8, 2024. https://healthpolicy.ucla.edu/sites/default/files/2023-08/tw_cba20.pdf

21. Vladimani, Sonia. Abundance mindset: why it's important and 8 ways to create it. Happiness.com. Accessed March 7, 2024. https://www.happiness.com/magazine/science-psychology/abundance-mindset/

22. Blanchfield, Theodora. How to shift from a scarcity mindset to an abundance mindset. Medically reviewed by Armeen Poor, MD. Verywellmind. March 24, 2022. Accessed March 7, 2024. https://www.verywellmind.com/how-to-shift-from-a-scarcity-mindset-to-an-abundance-mindset-5220862

23. Enhancing Rural Community Capacity, by Community-Development. July 12, 2019. Accessed March 8, 2024. https://community-development.extension.org/asset-mapping-a-quick-overview-and-related-resources/

24. What is positive deviance? Positive Deviance Collaborative. Accessed March 7, 2024. https://positivedeviance.org/

25. Miller-McLemore, B. The Living Human Web: A Twenty-five Year Retrospective. Published April 25, 2018. Accessed March 8, 2024. https://www.semanticscholar.org/paper/The-Living-Human-Web%3A-A-Twenty-five-Year-Miller-McLemore/e33b958bdf446e14d2e590f3f43bd8402d83d265

26. Exploring system failure: what is it and what do we know about it? Europe: Is the System Broken?, June 14, 2019, pp. 3-6 (4 pages) Accessed March 6, 2024. https://www.jstor.org/stable/resrep21475.4.

27. Meltdown: Why our systems fail and what we can do about it. Leadership Now. March 12, 2018. Accessed March 6, 2024. https://www.leadershipnow.com/leadingblog/2018/03/meltdown_why_our_systems_fail.html

28. Mambrol, Nasrullah. Structuralism. March 20, 2016. Accessed March 6, 2024. https://literariness.org/2016/03/20/structuralism/

29. Structuralism. https://en.wikipedia.org/wiki/Structuralism Accessed March 6, 2024.

3. Who We Are: Roles and Responsibilities

The transformative Rosenwald School project built more than 5000 schools, stores, and teachers homes between 1917 and 1932 to educate more than 700,000 Black children in the US South over four decades. The project was the result of the partnership between Julius Rosenwald, the Jewish-American part-owner and president of Sears, Roebuck and Company, and Booker T. Washington, a Black educator, philanthropist, leader, and president of the Black university, Tuskegee Institute.[30,31]

30. Rosenwald School. Wikipedia. Updated July 5, 2023. https://en.wikipedia.org/wiki/Rosenwald_School

31. Solender, Michael J. Inside the Rosenwald Schools. March 30, 2021. https://www.smithsonianmag.com/history/how-rosenwald-schools-shaped-legacy-generation-black-leaders-180977340/

32. Bennett, Neil et al. Who Had Medical Debt in the United States? 19% of U.S. Households Could Not Afford to Pay for Medical Care Right Away. U.S. Census Bureau. April 7, 2021. Https://www.census.gov/library/stories/2021/04/who-had-medical-debt-in-united-states.html

12. Viverette, Emily Bennett. Building Bridges: Integrating Community Engagement Skills into Clinical Pastoral Education at Atrium Health Wake Forest Baptist. (Hood Theological Seminary, DMin Project) Salisbury, NC, 2022. Accessed February 22, 2024

4. For the Good of the Hive: Community Engagement

33. Proverbs 27:18, Holy Bible, King James Version.

34. North Carolina Baptist Hospital: 100 Years of Caring, A Place of Healing and Teaching. Atrium Health Wake Forest Baptist. Accessed February 19, 2024. Baptist. https://www.wakehealth.edu/about-us/centennial

35. North Carolina Baptist Hospital: A House of Healing Celebrates 100 Years. Updated 2023. Accessed February 19, 2024. https://www.wakehealth.edu/about-us/centennial/a-house-of-healing

36. Annual of the North Carolina Baptist State Convention. Richmond Press: Richmond, VA, 1921. pp. 122-123.

37. The Moravian Church. Updated 2023. Accessed February 19, 2024. https://www.moravian.org/2018/07/a-brief-history-of-the-moravian-church/

38. Jones, L. Gregory. Christian Social Innovation: Renewing Wesleyan Witness. 2016. Accessed February 19, 2024. Pp 5-6.

8. James, Julia. Nonprofit Hospitals' Community Benefit Requirements. Health Affairs. February 25, 2016. Accessed July 10, 2024. https://www.healthaffairs.org/content/briefs/nonprofit-hospitals-community-benefit-requirements#:~:text=Under%20the%20%22community%20benefit%22%20standard%2C%20spending%20that%20promotes,determining%20what%20activities%20and%20services%20constituted%20community%20benefit.

12. Viverette, Emily Bennett. Building Bridges: Integrating Community Engagement Skills into Clinical Pastoral Education at Atrium Health Wake Forest Baptist. (Hood Theological Seminary, DMin Project) Salisbury, NC, 2022. Accessed February 19, 2024. Pp 14-15.

39. The Story of Stone Soup. Accessed July 11, 2024. https://www.learningtogive.org/sites/default/files/handouts/Story_Stone_Soup.pdf

40. Stone Soup. Accessed March 29, 2024. https://en.wikipedia.org/wiki/Stone_Soup

5. Nailing Jello to the Wall: Measuring the Impact of Chaplain Managers

41. Damen, Annelieke et al. Examining the Association Between Chaplain Care and Patient Experience. Journal of Patient Experience. April 19, 2020. https://www.ncbi.nlm.nih.gov/pmc/articles/PMC7786773/

42. Lichter, David A. Studies Show Spiritual Care Linked to Better Health Outcomes. Health Progress. Catholic Health Association of the US. March-April 2013. https://www.chausa.org/docs/default-source/health-progress/f761c4147687414ba9b12cabb8da03 4b1

12. Viverette, Emily Bennett. Building Bridges: Integrating Community Engagement Skills into Clinical Pastoral Education at Atrium Health Wake Forest Baptist. (Hood Theological Seminary, DMin Project) Salisbury, NC, 2022. Pp 18-20, 68, 72-75, 77-78, 105-115. Accessed February 22, 2024.

43. Social Determinants of Health for Rural People. Rural Health Information Hub (RHIHub). Updated 12/11/2023.

6. Hospital Closures Threaten Patient Access to Care as Hospitals Face a Range of Rising Pressures. American Hospital Association. September 8, 2022. https://www.aha.org/press-releases/2022-09-08-new-aha-report-finds-rural-hospital-closures-threaten-patient-access-care

7. Condon, Alan. States with the most rural hospital closures. Becker's Healthcare: Hospital CFO Report. November 28, 2023. Accessed July 12, 2024. https://www.beckershospitalreview.com/finance/states-with-the-most-rural-hospital-closures.html

44. McCloskey, Joe. "Atrium Health Wake Forest Baptist Reports Record-Setting $767.5 Million in Community Benefits in 2022." Atrium Health Wake Forest Baptist. November 15, 2023. https://newsroom.wakehealth.edu/news-releases/2023/11/atrium-health-wake-forest-baptist-reports-record-setting-community-benefits-in-2022

STUDIES ASSOCIATING CHAPLAIN CARE WITH GREATER PATIENT/FAMILY SATISFACTION WITH HOSPITAL CARE

Astrow, A.B. et al. Spiritual needs and perception of quality of care and satisfaction with care in hematology/medical oncology patients: a multicultural assessment. J Pain Symptom Manage [Internet]. 2018; 55:56–64. e1 doi:10.1016/j.jpainsymman.2017.08.009. https://pubmed.ncbi.nlm.nih.gov/28842220/

Clark, P.A., Drain, M., Malone, M.P. Addressing patients' emotional and spiritual needs. Jt Comm J Qual Saf. 2003;29:659–70. https://pubmed.ncbi.nlm.nih.gov/14679869/

Daaleman, T.P., Williams, C.S., Hamilton, V.L., Zimmerman, S. Spiritual care at the end of life in long-term care. Med Care [Internet]. 2008;46:85–91. https://oce.ovid.com/article/00005650-200801000-00013/HTML

Williams, J.A. et al. Attention to inpatients' religious and spiritual concerns: predictors and association with patient satisfaction. J Gen Intern Med [Internet]. 2011;26:1265–71. https://link.springer.com/article/10.1007/s11606-011-1781-y

6. Anglers and Bakers: Core Competencies and Skills

45. Atrium Health Wake Forest Baptist website. Diversity, Ethics, and Inclusion: Our Culture Commitments video. Accessed July 17, 2024. https://www.wakehealth.edu/about-us/inclusion-and-diversity

46. Healthy People 2030, U.S. Department of Health and Human Services, Office of Disease Prevention and Health Promotion. Accessed January 9, 2024, from https://health.gov/healthypeople/objectives-and-data/social-determinants-health.

9. Ridenhour, Adam. Beyond Clinical Specificity: A Model of Chaplaincy and Clinical Spiritual Care within the Shifting Paradigm of Population Health. 2022. Dissertation, Duke University Divinity School. Accessed March 6, 2024. Page 15. https://dukespace.lib.duke.edu/items/040bae67-d878-455a-8ccf-f739fdee8f00

47. Common Qualifications and Competencies for Professional Chaplains. Board of Chaplaincy Certification, Inc., an affiliate of APC. August 2023. Accessed July 18, 2024. https://www.apchaplains.org/bcci-site/becoming-certified/common-qualifications-and-competencies/

12. Viverette, Emily Bennett. Building Bridges: Integrating Community Engagement Skills into Clinical Pastoral Education at Atrium Health Wake Forest Baptist. (Hood Theological Seminary, DMin Project) Salisbury, NC, 2022. Accessed January 10, 2024

7. The Cup That Runneth Over: Challenges, Lessons, The Future

48. Alpert, Abby et al. Origins of the Opioid Crisis and Its Enduring Impacts. National Institutes of Health (NIH) National Library of Medicine. November 13, 2021. Accessed July 18, 2024. https://www.ncbi.nlm.nih.gov/pmc/articles/PMC9272388/

49. Eugenics and Scientific Racism fact sheet. National Institutes of Health (NIH) National Human Genome Research Institute. Updated May 18, 2022. Accessed July 18, 2024. https://www.genome.gov/about-genomics/fact-sheets/Eugenics-and-Scientific-Racism

50. COVID Data Tracker. Centers for Disease Control and Prevention (CDC). February 23, 2024. Accessed March 12, 2024. https://covid.cdc.gov/covid-data-tracker/#datatracker-home.

51. Bambino, Dan et al. Disproportionate Impact of COVID-19 on Racial and Ethnic Minority Groups in the United States: a 2021 Update. NIH. Oct. 13, 2021. Accessed March 12, 2024. https://www.ncbi.nlm.nih.gov/pmc/articles/PMC8513546/

52. Gillespie, Claire. Why Comorbidities Are a Risk Factor for Developing Severe COVID-19. Medically reviewed by Kashif J. Piracha, MD. Health.com. Updated October 9, 2022. Accessed March 12, 2024. https://www.health.com/condition/infectious-diseases/coronavirus/comorbidities-meaning-covid

53. Understanding the Opioid Epidemic. Centers for Disease Control and Prevention (CDC). Last reviewed August 8, 2023. Accessed April 17, 2024. https://www.cdc.gov/overdose-prevention/about/understanding-the-opioid-overdose-epidemic.html?CDC_AAref_Val=https://www.cdc.gov/opioids/basics/epidemic.html

54. Paris, Julia and Rowley, Caitlin. The economic impact of the opioid epidemic. Brookings. April 17, 2023. Accessed April 18, 2024. https://www.brookings.edu/articles/the-economic-impact-of-the-opioid-epidemic/

55. The High Price of the Opioid Crisis, 2021: Increasing access to treatment can reduce costs. The Pew Charitable Trusts. August 27, 2021. Accessed May 3, 2024. https://www.pewtrusts.org/en/research-and-analysis/data-visualizations/2021/the-high-price-of-the-opioid-crisis-2021

56. Luo, Feijun, Li, Mengyao, and Florence, Curtis. State-Level Economic Costs of Opioid Use Disorder and Fatal Opioid Overdose—United States, 2017. CDC Centers for Disease Control and Prevention. April 16, 2021. Accessed May 3, 2024. https://www.cdc.gov/mmwr/volumes/70/wr/mm7015a1.htm

57. Aboulenein, Ahmed. Opioid crisis cost U.S. nearly 1.5 trillion in 2020—congressional report. Reuters USA. September 28, 2022. Accessed May 3, 2024. https://www.reuters.com/world/us/opioid-crisis-cost-us-nearly-15-trillion-2020-congressional-report-2022-09-28/

58. Koh, Howard and Feldscher, Karen. What led to the opioid crisis—and how to fix it. Harvard School of Public Health. February 9, 2022. Accessed April 17, 2024. https://www.hsph.harvard.edu/news/features/what-led-to-the-opioid-crisis-and-how-to-fix-it/

59. More Than 40 Percent of Americans Know Someone Who Died of Drug Overdose; 13 Percent Say Deaths Have Disrupted Their Lives. Rand. February 21, 2024. Accessed February 22, 2024. https://www.rand.org/news/press/2024/02/21.html

60. Shipley, Alishiah. Opioid Crisis Affects All Americans, Rural and Urban. US Department of Agriculture (USDA). January 11, 2018. Accessed July 18, 2024. https://www.usda.gov/media/blog/2018/01/11/opioid-crisis-affects-all-americans-rural-and-urban

61. Underlying Medical Conditions Associated with Higher Risk for Severe COVID-19: Information for Healthcare Professionals. Centers for Disease Control and Prevention (CDC). Updated February 9, 2023. Accessed March 12, 2024. https://www.cdc.gov/coronavirus/2019-ncov/hcp/clinical-care/underlyingconditions.html

9. Ridenhour, Adam. Beyond Clinical Specificity: A Model of Chaplaincy and Clinical Spiritual Care within the Shifting Paradigm of Population Health. 2022. Dissertation, Duke University Divinity School. Accessed March 6, 2024. Page 15. https://dukespace.lib.duke.edu/items/040bae67-d878-455a-8ccf-f739fdee8f00

About the Authors

Rev. Graylin Carlton graduated from Foothills Christian College with a Bachelor of Christian Ministry and holds a Master of Ministry from Piedmont International University. He completed a unit of Level I CPE and a two-year CPE residency at Atrium Health Wake Forest Baptist Hospital. Graylin is an ordained Baptist minister and pastor of Oak Grove Missionary Church in Walkertown, NC. He also served as the evening chaplain at the Winston-Salem Rescue Mission before accepting the role of Staff Chaplain–Transitional Care at Atrium Health Wake Forest Baptist Hospital main campus. He loves living out his faith through caring for the needs of others by working in the trenches of community chaplaincy.

Rev. Dianne Horton earned a B.A. from Salem College in Sociology with a minor in Religion. She achieved the Master of Divinity Degree from Wake Forest University School of Divinity with the distinguished honor of receiving the John Thomas and Dorothy Porter Award for Vocational Formation and Community Ministry. A Board-certified chaplain with the Association of Professional Chaplains, she completed a two-year residency in Clinical Pastoral Education with a Pastoral Care Specialty in the Department of Chaplaincy and Pastoral Education, Division of Faith and Health Ministries at Wake Forest Baptist Health. She enjoys the freedom and flexibility of her role that allows her to engage in the sacred work of developing proactive means to improve the health of communities.

Rev. Dr. Adam Ridenhour is a graduate of Catawba College (B.A.), Wake Forest University School of Divinity (M.Div.), Wake Forest University Graduate School (M.A.), and Duke Divinity School (D.Min.). He is a Licensed Clinical Mental Health Counselor (LCMHC), a National Certified Counselor (NCC), and a Board-certified Chaplain (BCC) through the Association of Professional Chaplains. Adam is an ordained minister and endorsed chaplain affiliated with the Cooperative Baptist Fellowship. He enjoys the creativity and freedom of the FaithHealth work to accompany others through the complexities of health and wholeness.

Rev. Dr. Emily Viverette is an ordained minister in the Christian Church (Disciples of Christ). She holds a B.S. from Elon University, M.Div from Vanderbilt University, and D.Min from Hood Theological Seminary. She is also a Certified Educator via Association of Clinical Pastoral Education (ACPE, Inc). In her work to develop educational programming that advances the mission of FaithHealth, she is passionate about the ways in which faith communities, faith-based agencies, chaplains, and clergy can collaborate to improve health in their communities, particularly in rural settings.

Melanie Raskin is an award-winning writer, primarily in the health care and public health arenas. With a background in radio news, public relations, and marketing communications, her expertise includes writing articles and feature stories, websites and eblasts, video and audio scripts, online learning, press releases, slogans, and product names. Also a fiction writer with a number of publication credits and honors, she has a B. A. from the University of North Carolina–Chapel Hill, specializing in writing. While she has won many accolades, the greatest reward is partnering with smart, dedicated people to ensure readers find meaning in the content and are empowered to make a positive change.